I dedicate this book to all the nurses during 2020, this year has been so tough for us all, but we will remain strong and resilient, and we have become stronger nurses for the future. Thank you.

The events in this book occurred in 2020, all names of the patients and staff members I encountered, have been anonymized to maintain confidentiality

Contents

Chapter 1: Return to the ward
Chapter 2: Accident and Emergency
Chapter 3: Secret tapes and Groundhog Day
Chapter 4: The stroke ward
Chapter 5: Return to the medical ward
Chapter 6: isolation
Chapter 7: Community panic
Chapter 8: Community terror
Chapter 9: The battle continues
Chapter 10: Winter Pressure
Chapter 11 Look to the future
Chapter 12: The calm before the storm
Chapter 13: A reflection for the future
Chapter 14: A letter from my brother
Chapter 15: top tips for nurse's post-2020

Chapter 1: Return to the ward.

Throughout 2019 I worked as an actor in New York, working in different productions such as cats and Pinocchio. I lived in a studio apartment in Manhattan with my nephew Harry. After working as a rotational nurse in busy wards it felt refreshing coming to New York and returning to my work as an actor. I worked long hours as an actor, rehearsing my lines, and completing twenty shows a week in front of hundreds of people. At the end of my day, I would collect my nephew Harry from the playschool, return home to cook dinner and speak to my family via skype in the UK, to catch up on daily events.

On my day's off I would attend the cinema or go to dinner with my fellow actors and take my nephew Harry to popular amusements in the Manhattan area. In my time as a nurse, I always had to rush to work and return home quickly. During my time in New York, I would drink my hot chocolate each morning with a bagel. During my break from the theatre, I would go ice skating or take a run through the town. Working as an actor and performing in front of a crowd gave me such an amazing buzz. However, my time as a nurse, and caring for people, and making a difference in their lives, left me with a sense of satisfaction that I was making a difference in the world.

For over eight years, I was torn between choosing between my career as a nurse and actor. In 2020, my life was about to turn upside down, and I was about to recommence my nursing journey during one of the hardest times for medical professionals in history.

In March 2020 I returned to visit my parents in Yorkshire, my Mother worked as a librarian at the local library, whilst my Father was now retired from his job as a teacher.

As I returned to my childhood home, I found it increasingly difficult entering my old bedroom, which I shared with my brother Michael, who passed away eight years previously. All of Michael's belongings, his books, clothes and pictures, were stacked neatly in boxes. Whilst his bed and his office desk were left untouched. Being back in the bedroom reminded me of all the time I spent supporting my brother during his cancer illness, caring for him, staying at his bedside, and comforting him during his illness. I also remembered the happier times we shared, gazing at the stars through our telescope, staying up until midnight to watch our scary movies, and singing our favorite songs on our karaoke machine.

I had planned only a short visit to the UK with Harry, it felt wonderful spending time with my parents. We would watch the news of the reported 'coronavirus' and my Father would laugh at the internet footage of people rushing to get toilet roll. At the time we were in denial, believing that the coronavirus was nothing but a mere media storm.

During my visit to see my parents, we spent time with each other including going to theme parks, going out to restaurants together or seeing our favorite film. In the afternoon I would walk with Harry along the cobbled Yorkshire country roads.

We had heard news reports about the coronavirus in the media for a few weeks, and then at 5 pm, we sat in front of the television to watch the Boris Johnson conference. We looked on in fear as Boris announced the lockdown, explaining that schools were closed, and the enforcement of new guidelines, staying at home as much as possible and only going out once a day for exercise.

Immediately I thought about my future in New York, how and when could I go back if they close the borders? What will I do to support myself and Harry financially? Could I cope with living with my parents with all the memories I held of caring for my brother through his illness?
The next few days were very unusual, I felt like a caged animal trapped at home. I almost felt guilty about going outside. As I walked down the long country road to the town centre, my heart would pound as soon as a person would come near. I felt suffocated in the mask as I walked into the Tesco garage. I immediately became frustrated, watching as people failed

to follow the 2-metre distance rule. I could see an old friend in the distance pull up in the car in a haze of anxiety as I made my way home.

As I arrived back home, I changed my clothes and sterilized my hands, I felt contaminated.

I looked on in sadness as my parents cancelled their forty years anniversary cruise to Egypt.

"Both you and Harry can stay here for as long as you want, I know this is a difficult time, I don't think you will be going home anytime soon," Mum warned

"I love the theatre, I've made so many friends, completed so many plays I finally feel happy and now this has happened." I began.

"Well I feel it will be nice to have you and Harry around for a while, it's nice to hear the sound of a child laughing in the house," my Mum smiled. It was then that my Mother placed the lasagna on the table, and we enjoyed our meal together.

I thought about my fellow colleagues at the hospital, wondering what life was like for them on the wards during the pandemic. I suspected that the staff would be following strict social distancing duties, whilst carrying on their duties, with fear, hiding behind a heated mask and gloves.

I became concerned during the first couple of weeks of the lockdown, reading about the lack of PPE equipment available in the NHS, the devastating fatal deaths of NHS staff, who were unable to obtain protective equipment. I looked on in sadness and distress at the high rate of care home residents who contracted the virus, and the battle their families began in a desperate attempt to see them.

That evening, I decided to ring the previous sister I worked with on the Stroke ward, Sister Diana. Sister Diana was one of the most caring, hard-working nurses I had ever worked with. Sister Diana would ensure that she knew the name of all the patients on the ward and would leave at 9 pm after staying over to complete her notes.

"Hi, I just wanted to check how you are doing? I'm back in Yorkshire for a few months, I know it's a hard time."

"Well Chris it has been really difficult, we have to wear our masks all day, we are more short-staffed than we have ever been, the hospital chiefs are threatening to close the ward and move us to high dependencies wards. We are all exhausted and overworked, do you think you could come back and help us?" she asked.

"Well it's been a long time now since I've worked on the wards, I'm not sure I would know what to do!"

"You will be fine; say you will think about it?" Diana pleaded.

"Ok," I lied. I found nursing a difficult and stressful occupation, during a pandemic would heighten the difficulties of the job.

Over the next few weeks in lockdown, I found it so hard looking after my nephew trying to entertain him. Over the first few weeks of lockdown, Harry had watched almost every Disney film, colored in twenty coloring books, climbed the tall oak trees in our garden, and went on over fifty bike rides a week.

Harry had really struggled to adjust to life in the UK and his sleeping routine had completely changed, he struggled to sleep and missed the food from the US.

As I completed daily exercise, I was constantly reminded of my time in the NHS. Posters titled 'join the NHS' and billboards which read 'stay home and protect the NHS' helped me to realize the important job I had as a nurse, and the terrifying effect the coronavirus had on the staff and hospital sector.

In looking at my financial situation and in watching the 'return to work' NHS advertisement, I decided that I wanted to rejoin the NHS on the bank system as a temporary staff member, to help my colleagues, I felt I had a duty as a qualified nurse to help my colleagues.

As I sat with my Mum during a curry night, I decided to reveal my plans. "Mum I've thought about it a lot and I want to return to the NHS as a bank nurse working on different wards."

"Are you sure Chris? What about the risks to yourself to us, I mean your Father has asthma, we would have to separate from each other," Mum warned.

"Well, I can have my own cutlery, wash my laundry separately, and watch movies in a different room." I offered.

"Well I just hope you are making the right decision," Mum warned.

The following day I contacted the Yorkshire temporary staffing service and collected my bright blue nursing uniform. That evening I made my cheese sandwiches, prepared my nursing notebook and ironed my uniform ready for the next day. In my pocket, I had three sanitizer gels and attached my fob watch to the front of my nursing blazer. As I rested my head on the pillow that night, I felt like I was about to enter a battle.

Chapter 2: Accident and Emergency chaos

I awoke the next morning at 5:30 am to the sound of the bluebirds in the oak trees chirping. I was nervous and shaking as I ran downstairs, my mind was racing as I thought about my day shift, and the possible tasks I would have to undertake. I quickly ran down the spiral staircase and ate a few slices of my toast, and only managed a few sips of my green tea. Leaving the hospital for over a year made it very difficult going back, especially in a worldwide pandemic. I walked down the cobbled path nervously, as my heart began to pound through my chest. The greatest hits of Queen on my iPod and breathing in the fresh frosty air, helped me to feel refreshed in the morning.

I arrived at the hospital at 6:30 am, my hands were trembling, and my heart skipped a beat. I observed bank nurses, lined up outside of the nursing Manager's office, waiting to be allocated to different wards. Sister Debbie walked over to me, "Nice to see you, Chris, I hope you enjoyed your break! You will be in an accident and emergency today." she smiled.

I gulped and forced a smile, of all the wards I worked on I found accident and Emergency the hardest ward to work on. As I reached the ward, I saw a basket filled with masks. As soon as I wore the mask, I could feel my face heat up, I instantly felt uncomfortable. I was met by the ward sister Sally Betson, an authoritative, prompt, hard-working nurse.

"Hi Chris, today you will be in charge of cubicles one to six," she said robotically. The ward was shaped into a fishbowl, with the nursing staff and doctors sitting at their station in the middle of the ward. Around the station were hospital trolleys, and only a few patients were on the ward. As I entered, I witnessed an elderly man wearing a cap holding a bloody bandage on his head. Then I witnessed a man and wife holding hands, nervously, waiting for the results of their scan, whilst a teenage girl shouted at a nurse having been admitted following fracturing her leg on the ice rink. As I stood around, I watched the nurse's running around the ward, rushing to complete their tasks, answering buzzers, and nervously writing their notes before the end of the shift.

My first patient in bay one was Hayley Williams, a ninety-year-old lady. Hayley was admitted after being found wandering in the streets at midnight. Hayley lived alone, and it was discovered that she had over a hundred cats filling each room in the house. Hayley was very confused and had displayed unusual behavior ever since her husband passed away a year previously. Hayley's hair was red, curly, and wild, she wore a bright blue nightgown, and was very defensive when I spoke to her.

Hello, Hayley, I am your nurse Chris I am here to help you." I smiled.

"I don't need your help!" she smiled.

"I am here if you need a nurse," I offered.

"Well Carry on Simon, help someone else, I am very happy I do not need any help."

The plan for Hayley was to complete a memory test and refer to the memory clinic if she scored poorly, and I had to liaise with the mental health team who were due to assess her.

Suddenly the ambulance team admitted two men, a man wearing a suit, who was admitted following a collapse in his kitchen before work, and the second patient was Sally Evans, a forty-two-year-old lady, admitted with chest pain. I quickly set up their beds pace, setting up their bedside table and passed their buzzers by their bedside,

I walked into John's cubicle and completed the ECG and took bloods. I could see the fear and look of terror on his face, as I took his observations.

"I am so sorry I'm just so nervous, my Father died of a heart attack at fifty and I'm worried. I'm a finance consultant, and I can't really afford to be off for even a day," he warned. I noticed that John's observations were in the normal range, but his blood sugar reading was high.

"John, your observations are in the normal parameter, but your blood sugar is high, I will get Dr Cartmell to see you." I smiled.

I had been in the ward for less than an hour, and I already felt like I had never left. I walked over to Dr Cartmell and admired his work ethic, as he jumped up and attended to John following his low reading.

I then walked over to Sally Cartmell, who was being assessed by Doctor Wright, Sally sat in her Rugrat pajamas, "I feel like I'm going to die, I'm frightened, I feel sick she roared."

I watched as Doctor Wright assessed Sally's breathing rate with the stethoscope, and he discovered that she was possibly suffering from anxiety.

"Anxiety? That's all you keep saying, I want a second opinion, I need to see another doctor!" she roared.

"I can arrange that for you, Dr Wright," smiled.

"Quick Chris front door," Sally shouted. As I looked at the main door, I witnessed Hayley holding her bags, trying to get out.

"Open the doors, I want to go home. I hate it here!" she shouted.

"Please Hayley, come back to your bedside I will make you a warm cup of tea,"

"Go away Move!" She shouted.

"How about I give you a chocolate biscuit and a Jaffa cake,"

"Ok," Hayley smiled, completely changing her mood as she walked to her bedside. As I sat with Hayley that morning, I completed the memory test asking her to name the animals, complete simple sums, and recall basic facts. Hayley failed each question and showed that her memory was impaired, and the next step was to refer her to the memory clinic for further assessment for dementia.

I then sat in the nurse's office for my lunch break, I felt guilty on my break, thinking of all the tasks I had yet to complete. I felt relieved to take my mask off and looked on in fear in the mirror, noticing the red marks etched around my face. The two nurses in the office closed their eyes and were exhausted slouched on the sofa.

After my break, I observed how stressed Sister Sally was, there were five members of the public at the nurse's desk demanding a covid test, believing they displayed symptoms. Sister Sally stood with confidence, "if you feel you have symptoms, you need to call 111 and book a test, we are not able to facilitate tests in Accident and Emergency," she warned.

In the department, there was so much fear and panic in the eyes of the other healthcare workers on the nurse station, worried that they may have been exposed to the coronavirus.

As I walked back onto the ward, I now had two extra patients to look after. The first was seventy-nine-year-old Tom, who was admitted following an urgent referral from the GP, for an infection in his ulcerative legs. Tom was joined by his overpowering wife who would sit and cry hysterically.
The final patient was Ethel, a ninety-year-old lady admitted after having a fall at home, her face and arms were covered in bruises, but she smiled sweetly as she sat knitting a baby's cardigan.

I watched as Hayley smiled as she was being moved by the porters for further assessment at the general medical ward. Dr Cartmell then walked over to me, "John's results have come back, and we've just revealed that he is diabetic, he will be moving to the diabetic ward tomorrow, but he is very anxious so please monitor him," Dr Cartmell smiled.
I walked over to John and watched as tears rolled down his cheek, "I suspect the diabetic condition was caused by self-neglect. After my wife left me, I started drinking unhealthily and eating takeaways each night. Would you be able to help me look at adjusting my food options?" he asked.

"Of course, I will".

I then discussed with John healthy food options, and we discussed looking at him eating smaller food portions and substituting his sugary foods for alternative heavy snacks. I watched as the etched expression of fear changed in John's face and he was content, and I knew this was what I loved about my job.

I then walked over to Tom and Mary, as they sat arguing in his cubicle. John was dressed in red pajamas and had long black hair, whilst Mary was dressed in her pink fur dress. "Shut up Mary, let the gentlemen speak," he ushered.

"Tom I'm just going to complete the dressing on your legs if that's ok?"

I watched as Tom nodded his head. Suddenly Mary began to cry hysterically, "Oh Doctor, Doctor, he never listens to me he just says he doesn't love me, but I love him."

"It's ok Mary, would you like to go to the canteen and have a sandwich?" I offered. I watched as Mary walked away and I completed the dressing and looked on and marveled at how happy Tom was. Mary returned from the coffee shop more anxious than before and began to sob.

"Oh, doctor I'm so pleased you have looked after my husband, but please help me, I don't think he loves me anymore!" she screeched.

I walked over to Gretel and completed her observations which were all in the normal range. I booked a scan just to rule out any fracture following her fall. Gretel was a kind and gentle lady, and she loved being around people.

"It is so scary for Britain in the current pandemic. My mother lived through the Spanish flu, she lost two close friends who she befriended during the war, mum said life was never the same again. It's funny how much we take for granted, walking freely into a shop, sitting together with our friends, catching a movie. Now our lives are restricted, and we will have to learn to adapt, we must be resilient to get through this," she smiled.
"I agree I smiled.

My first day back in an accident and emergency was very hectic. There was so much fear on the ward for all staff and patients. I was exhausted, after running around the ward, and my face was left in deep red marks from wearing the mask all day. I went home and I was treated to a Yorkshire roast dinner from my mother, and collapsed onto the bed, contemplating on my first day back as a nurse.

Chapter 3: Secret tapes and Groundhog Day

The positive aspect of working as a nurse on the bank team was being able to pick and choose when I wanted to work. In the lockdown, I found it so difficult sitting at home, and desperately fighting to maintain the social distancing rules when venturing outside.

I received a call from Harry's nursery explaining that they felt I should come and collect him, due to a change in his behavior. As I walked up to the nursery, I was shocked when I observed Harry sitting in a ball pit hysterically crying.

"What happened? Why is Harry so upset?"

"Well he became angry at lunchtime, he ripped a huge section of wallpaper from the wall, he threw his lunch on the floor, we just feel he may prefer going home early today.

As I walked with Harry to the car, his breathing became more controlled and the tears were more controlled.

"What's wrong, why are you so upset?" I asked.

"I miss my home in New York, it's so boring here and we can't even go to the movies anymore!" he screeched,

"We will go back to New York after the virus has cleared, we just have to wait." I smiled. As I arrived home I watched as Harry fell asleep on the sofa, he was exhausted after a long day at nursery and struggled to adapt to his new life in the UK.

That evening I completed a task that I had put off for over five years. I had to organize my brother Michael's belongings, kept in the bedroom, closet and decided what I was going to keep and throw away.

As I walked up to the room, I took a deep breath as I began to put his belongings into the box. In the closet, I discovered several journals and medical textbooks that he had stored. Then I found a photo album filled with a collage of photos of the memories we shared through the years, from our graduation to our holiday to Florida, to the photo of the first mini that we saved for.

It was so hard returning home, revisiting memories I shared with my brother, living in New York helped me to escape my grief, returning home brought back so many memories, and made me miss the life I had before he passed away.

Then as I reached for the top shelf, I discovered three videotapes in a box, containing the self-made videos of his time in the USA during his years working as a student doctor.

I decided to spend the evening watching videos. Michael would make the videos as a diary of his life to reflect on his difficult times.

The first video showed Michael sitting in his apartment after a long shift, upset after failing his practical exam, and exhausted after three staff members called in sick. Michael then expressed he found it lonely in his apartment, as his other colleagues studying art degrees had more time to socialize whilst studying took up most of Michael's time. At the same time, I was studying for my acting degree, enjoying making new friends and travelling with my castmates. The parallels of how different our lives became apparent.

I then watched the second video of Michael travelling with his girlfriend Louise. I watched as they climbed the Rocky Mountains at the Grand Canyon. At the top of the cliff, he proposed to Louise as the sun started to set. Michael had kept his private life hidden from us, and It felt strange looking at a part of his life that he kept hidden away. In the next part of the video, I watched as he completed his skydive, in memory of our Grandad who died of dementia. I watched as he landed in an open field as his flat mates clapped, before surprising him with a multicolored cake with sparklers attached. As I looked through the cupboard, I found several other videos but realized I was not ready to watch them all.

The following morning, I arrived at the hospital, hoping to be placed in a different ward. I enjoyed being in Accident and Emergency, but I also enjoyed being on different wards. As I turned up to the sister's ward I was frustrated as Sister Rita stated I would be sent to Accident and Emergency. I felt like I was cursed, but it was my duty as a bank nurse to work on any ward I was assigned to.

I struggled to breathe efficiently under the visa, it was a barrier towards patients and to staff members. In the accident and emergency ward, each shift was different to the next, sometimes I would walk into a quiet ward environment, and then in the next shift, I would walk onto a chaotic ward. As I walked into the emergency department, I could hear the emergency buzzer ring, as the red lights began to flash. A Man at fifty years old, admitted with sepsis went into cardiac arrest. Suddenly I observed doctors, nurses, and healthcare assistants rushing towards the unresponsive patient. I stood around the bed and watched as a newly qualified nurse completed CPR, whilst the senior consultant shouted out instructions. After two other staff members completed compressions it was now my turn. I watched as the curly-headed consultant shouted instructions, 'slower, faster, mask, stop!" I could feel my hands trembling as I completed the compressions, there was no sign of breathing after five minutes. Ten minutes later the patient was declared dead.

After each cardiac arrest, we would have to write a report, and then join a huddle to discuss how what happened, and how we would improve in the next emergency.

I had been in the ward for only twenty minutes and felt so warm and uncomfortable under the mask. On the doors of the ward were posters, warning anyone with symptoms to return home and call 111. I felt constantly nervous throughout the shift, washing my hands constantly, always aware of infection prevention.

The sister on the ward was Kate, a self-centered Nurse who would never support colleagues and instead stand behind the desk talking to doctors. Sandra, the health care assistant I would work alongside, had over forty years of healthcare experience and was willing to help in every task. The other nurse on the ward Kelly was constantly on her phone and would not help any other staff members.

Today I was looking after patients in cubicles twenty-five to thirty, and I was near the exit away from the noise of the nurse's station.

My first patient was Mike, and an eighty-nine-year-old man admitted from a nursing home, the staff had struggled with his behavior and felt that he required further assessment. Mike had long grey curly hair which he refused to cut, he was very hostile and angry and would wave his stick to anyone who would walk past. In the next bed with thirty-eight-year-old Karen, who was waiting to be discharged following a minor car accident outside of the hospital. Opposite Karen with forty-five-year-old Louise who admitted herself following severe headaches at home. Next to Laura was Claudia, a sixty-five-year-old woman, admitted with an exacerbation in her COPD. Next to Claudia was Simon, a homeless man, admitted following the discovery of him having an epileptic fit in the street.

Kate admitted that for the final two hours of my shift I would be working in the intensive care unit with James, a sixty-nine-year-old man who had contracted Coronavirus. I was nervous but well prepared by a senior member of staff, to look after patients who contracted the virus.

I could see the fear in the faces of the staff, hidden begin their masks and visas, despite signs on the doors, members of the public would still turn up at the reception desk asking for covid tests. Staff were exhausted, trying to reach targets and admitting a record number of patients a day. It was such a tense environment and we felt trapped inside a bubble of fear and worry. I returned to the ward environment to help others, but nothing could prepare me for the fear and anxiety I felt.

I walked over to mike to give him his medication for the day. "Who are you?" he growled.
"I'm Chris, I'm your nurse today," I smiled.
"You can piss off, don't touch anything," He warned, closing his walking stick close to his chest.
"I'm here to help you. I have your medication," I explained. As I walked slowly towards Mike, he grabbed his stick and smashed it on the table, causing the jug of water to crash onto the floor. I called for Sara, the healthcare assistant, to help me. It was so difficult for a person living with dementia to cope in a ward environment with a high level of noise, the bright noise and different staff wearing brightly colored toys. We managed to help Mike calm down by providing him with a cup of tea. Sara had a patient and gentle manner and managed to engage Mike by talking about his life in the army.

I then observed how angry Karen was having stayed in the Accident and Emergency overnight.

"Nurse I really need to go home; I'm an accountant and I've got several new staff members in my team."

"We are just waiting for your tablets and then we can discharge you."

"If I am not discharged by 12 pm I am going to put in a complaint to the hospital board," She warned.

I then observed Louise holding her head in pain, crying out. I completed Louise's observation discovering that her heart rate was over 110 beats per minute and her temperature was very high.

"I have been having headaches now for over six months, but they have really intensified, I can't sleep, I can't concentrate, and my eyesight has been affected, I'm just so concerned as my mother had a brain tumor previously and it was inoperable, I just need answers," She warned. I assured Louise by consulting with the junior doctor, booking her in for a CT scan.

  I then observed the newly qualified nurse Hayley struggling in her section one to five, and she had a patient requiring an urgent ECG, whilst she had to help log roll her patient who was admitted from a care home.

At times it was so hard working in Accident and Emergency as a Newly qualified nurse. As a newly qualified nurse you are still developing in the learning phase as a nurse, but you often have to complete assessments on your own, whilst looking after patients with high levels of need, during times when the ward was often short-staffed. I helped Hayley through helping her with tasks attempting to offload the pressure on Hayley.

As I returned to my bay, I watched as a frightened Louise was being taken for her CT scan, I was now hopeful she would finally receive the answers she was hoping for. I then observed Simon sitting comfortably in the recliner chair, with several blankets wrapped around him. Simon had been living on the streets of London for over three years, after being thrown out of his home.

"Well Chris I must say coming to the hospital has been a lifesaver for me, I've had my first hot meal in years, a constant flow of refreshing water, for the past couple years the food I have eaten has been the scraps leftover in the bin." he smiled.

The doctors became concerned as following his hallucination he was observed talking to shadows on the walls. The doctors requested for Simon to have a mental health examination. Simon presented as weak and malnourished, he was now only seven stone and struggled with his mobility.

"Thank you for the blankets and warm food Chris, it's been so long since anyone has spoken to me, you have made me feel human again," he smiled. It was then that I knew this was the true essence of being a nurse, despite how hard nursing can sometimes be, the positive recognition from patients is the biggest reward.

I looked at the front door of the Accident and Emergency department and watched as an angry Karen stormed out of the ward, refusing to wait for her tablets. "I will be reporting the staff on this ward for gross negligence!" she shouted.

As I looked around the department, I noticed an atmosphere of chaos and tension in the ward. I watched as senior doctors sat at the nurse's station, discussing the possible surge in coronavirus cases and the impact on patients. Whilst the ward sister Kate was outside, encouraging people arriving for tests to go to the covid pods for tests. I then observed the fear on the faces of the patients wearing masks, concerned about the risks involved in contracting the virus.

I then observed Mike Sitting with his wife, a look of fear on his face. I observed Mike's wife Barbara sitting in her Fur coat, as a tear rolled down her cheek. "I feel like Mike's behavior is getting worse, he does not remember who I am," she cried.

"That's because you're a stranger, and I do not want to see you, please go away!" he begged. I watched as an unsteady Mike began to stand up, unsteadily, dropping his walking stick on the floor.

"Sit down!" Barbra shouted.

"No, I need to go home to see my mother," he shouted.

"Help," I shouted, as Mike became unsteady on his feet. Suddenly, two healthcare assistants, Shirley and Vicky came to my rescue, guiding Mike towards the bed.

I sat next to Mike as he regained his composure, "Where am I? All I want to do is go home, my parents will expect me home for tea at 5 pm." he cried. I watched as Mike nervously looked around the ward. Mike believed he was fifteen years old, everything about the ward, the noise, the fast-moving staff, the bleeping of the observation machines left him greatly confused. As I sat with Mike, I thought about the previous dementia specialist ward I worked on which had door sensors, less staff and dementia-friendly colors. The ward environment was not conducive for people living with dementia, and instead only increased anxiety and agitation. I then observed as the mental health team arrived, and completed the assessment for Mike, observing that he was now in the middle stages of dementia and required specialist dementia care.

I felt so tired walking around the department, it was a battle remembering to take a drink of water. That afternoon I walked into the side room and observed an upset Claudia crying.

"Well Chris it looks like I've been given my final warning, no more cigarettes or I'll hit the bucket," she smiled.

"How many do you smoke?" I asked.

"Sixty a day, it's my only comfort since the passing of my husband, it helps me whenever I feel depressed." she cried.

That afternoon I referred Claudia to the Age UK service, and to her local community center, she stated she missed human contact and wanted to be around other people.

As the twilight nurse came in, I had to go to the intensive care room to support Jack who was on a ventilator. I felt so uncomfortable in my visa mask and protective suit. Jack felt very weak and was taking sips of water but was responding well to treatment. Working in intensive care provided close observation of patients, and in my role, I had to complete observations every fifteen minutes and turn the patient, to protect against pressure sores. As I sat in intensive care, I thought about Michael and how difficult he would find the lockdown. I could imagine he would defy the rules and travel to the beach every day. The lockdown had forced me for the first time in eight years, to confront my fear of living alone. I had battled so hard to come to terms with the loss of my brother.

It was so difficult after my shift to unwind in the lockdown. In my days in the past, I would go to the cinema, a drive to London, or a trip to the shops, but now I feel trapped in a lockdown imprisoned in my own house.

I continued to watch the home movies he made, finding out so much about him. I watched him travel to Disneyland on the trip away after his first year at college with Samantha. I watched as he enjoyed the tower of terror and put his fingers in the imprints at the movie studio. I observed as they returned to Michael's luxury apartment, he shared a luxury hotel with a swirl pool, a golden spiral staircase and a games room.

My weekends prior to the coronavirus were filled with fun and relaxation, going out to dinner, going to the cinema and visiting friends. Now I was fearful to go out, I was worried others would not maintain social distancing and I would be at risk.

I walked with Harry to Cover beach, with our Labrador puppy Cody. Harry would ask constant questions about Michael, asking what he enjoyed doing and what he did as a doctor. Coming back to England was a big adjustment to Harry, and our house was surrounded by pictures of Michael, the father he never met.

When we arrived at Cove beach, I smiled as I breathed in the cool brisk morning air. I walked along the soft sand overlooking the crystal blue water, In the distance was a rocky mountain. For so many years both I and Simon, would swim to the mountain and climb on it before diving back into the sea. As we walked along the beach, I let Harry hold the lead after he pleaded to throughout the journey. A minute after walking Cody Harry let go of the lead, and I frantically ran after Cody as he dived into the sea. At only ten weeks old Cody struggled to keep his head up. Harry began to cry, I struggled into the water and managed to grab a shivering Cody out of the water. There were so many memories I conjured being on the beach with my brother, having a party around the campfire with our friends after school, playing badminton on the beach, swimming in the sea at midnight with our friends whilst looking up into the stars.

As I walked home with Harry I glanced at my mobile, observing that I had over a dozen messages from my friends in New York, expressing their anguish at the closing of the theatres, suddenly their acting work had dried up. I began to wonder when I would ever return to acting, and I wondered if I would have to extend my stay in the UK as a nurse, to support myself financially.

I went home that evening, and my mother had prepared a luxurious roast dinner with turkey and roast turkey drizzled in warm velvet gravy. I watched as a soaked Cody lay beside the hot fire. As I watched my parents and Harry sitting around the table laughing, I realized I was in the best place, with my family, all together and no longer alone.

Chapter 4: The stroke ward

As I returned to the nursing manager's office at the hospital, I was delighted that I was sent to the stroke ward. I worked on the stroke ward for over a year as a newly qualified nurse, and I felt like I was back with my family. Sister Diana was my previous mentor, as a student nurse and helped to teach me the basics of being a nurse, and I always attempted to model her communication methods, she was so kind, caring and compassionate, knowing the names of all the patients on the ward and caring for both the physical and mental wellbeing of patients. Nurse Ross was forty-three and originally worked as a nurse in the Philippines for over twenty years. Whilst nurse Katyanna was a kind-hearted nurse but was known as one of the laziest nurse's in the trust, constantly barking orders at staff to offload work she didn't want to.

"Oh Chris, I must say, it's wonderful to see you even in such difficult circumstances, thank you for helping us," Diana smiled before embracing me tightly.

I took a deep breath as I put on the mask, I instantly felt uncomfortable dressed in scrubs, and struggled to talk through the suffocating visa. Sister Diana introduced me to my patients. In the side room, one was ninety-one-year-old Derek admitted with bowel cancer. A kind and gentle man who fought in World War 2, and his room was filled with pictures.

In the bay, I met the three patients I was supporting.

The first patient, Louise, was admitted following a stroke and had recently qualified as a dentist. The stroke had affected her artistic abilities, and the ward staff were warned to not let her boyfriend who she split up with onto the ward.

The second patient was eighty-year-old Frances, who was admitted following a worsening of her dementia condition, having experienced a left-sided stroke two years earlier. Frances had struggled at home leaving the door open and paying money to people pretending to do 'jobs' at her house. Frances' neighbor reported her behavior to the social services department leading to her admission to hospital. The third patient was Jane, a sixty-eight-year-old lady, who lived who was admitted following a full stroke, but due to her depression, she was reluctant to engage in any therapy.

In the second side room was Milton who was admitted after the district nurse discovered that he was hiding his medication and forgetting to take them.

I realized that the ward environment post-pandemic was so different to the ward environment before. It was so unusual to have no visitors on the ward; the ward was covered in social distancing signs and keep out signs. The nurses and healthcare assistants were confined to their own bays.

Already I was in the ward for only a half an hour, and I had to run to the staff room for a sip of water, I was so weak and tired.

The morning was so busy, Derek struggled to take his tablets, as he was so physically tired, he took ten minutes to take tablets. I had to actively encourage Louise and Jane to take their tablets. Having a stroke can affect processing verbal messages in the brain, so I had to guide Louise and Jane by holding the tablets and cup of water in their hands.

Frances became very angry and threw the tablets at me as she believed I had disturbed her from her sleep.

Completing the personal care on the ward was so difficult, as nurses we would have to use hoists, standing aids and physically support the patients to sit up as the stroke affected their fine motor skills.

I worked with Helen, a health care assistant with over forty years of health care experience. As we supported Louise with a wash, I felt so warm under the mask, it was so hard to communicate with patients underneath a mask, I felt so restricted. We watched as Louise cried as we hoisted her into her rise and recliner chair. Each morning Helen would place a colored pencil in her hand and help guide Louise to draw on the page to encourage movement. On Louise's table was her graduation certificate from completing her dentistry course, and another picture showed her swimming in the crystal blue ocean.

Jane was very reluctant to engage in wash and dressing and cried into her pillow. I watched as Helen sat next to her stroking her hand, and offered her a warm cup of tea to help encourage her to engage. Helen's kind and gentle approach encouraged patients to take part in stroke therapy. Slowly, Jane was happy to take part in washing and dressing, and as we hoisted her into the chair, Helen provided extra care to her, brushing her hair, applying the moisturizer and helping her to take the mouthwash. We felt privileged in helping patients who required full support.

That morning I assisted Derek with his cooked breakfast. He required assistance with cutting up food, and I noticed how positive he was despite his terminal prognosis.

"It's not often you see male nurses; did you always want to be a nurse?"

"I trained originally as an actor; I've lived in New York for a few hours working as a theatre actor. I suppose I'm here because of the pandemic, it's my duty to return and help.

How are you coping, Derek? I know the chemotherapy treatment can be quite grueling."

"Well, the doctor explained to me yesterday that I only have six months left to live. I thought instead of being depressed and focusing on the negatives I would plan. So, I called my wife Samantha and we planned a spa retreat in Florida, and we are spending two weeks in Vegas, the place we met. I want to enjoy the time I have left; I just hope the restrictions are lifted," he smiled.

It was so encouraging to see how brave Derek was being despite the diagnosis. It suddenly dawned on me how difficult it was for patients living with cancer in the pandemic, with delays in treatment and so much uncertainty for the future.

As I walked to the nurse's station, I noticed a man in his early thirties standing by the ward door, in a blue checkered shirt holding flowers in his hands. "Hello sir, I was wondering if you could give these to my girlfriend Louise, I know she's not talking to me." He sighed.

"I'm really sorry but flowers are no longer allowed on the ward," I warned. It was then that Louise's boyfriend passed a note into my head to give to Louise. As I walked over to Louise, I passed her the note and she turned her head in defiance refusing to look at it. I observed how Louise became more depressed during the shift, I encouraged her to engage in therapy, explaining that even a short session with the physiotherapists will make such a difference.

As I went into the physio gym, I observed Jane sitting on the plinth with Michael and Anne the physiotherapists, sitting at her side keeping her balanced. As Michael stood in front of Jane and held onto her hands, she repeatedly said no whenever Michael asked her to tap her feet. Having a stroke is such a traumatic experience and treating depression can be just as important as treating the stroke.

Minutes later, Jane's Grand Daughter Anna, arrived visiting from Australia with her chocolate Labrador Poppy. Suddenly I could see a light in Jane, and she cried with happiness. With Anna watching in the distance I watched as Jane was able to tap her feet and managed to stand with minimal support, proving that encouragement and being positive helped to encourage progress.

It was very difficult to support Milton and Frances who were living with dementia, both struggled on the ward with loud noises, numerous staff members walking past and flashing lights. Milton became very agitated in the afternoon, and he stormed into the female bay, throwing his bottle of water at a startled female patient.

"You should look after your patients properly. This is disgraceful, I thought you were meant to protect patients!" Dawn shouted as I passed her towels. As I walked out of the bay, Sister Diana was instantly able to diffuse the situation. Diana took Milton by the hand and guided him toward the nurse's station, he sat on a chair whilst Diane gave him a set of folders asking if he could file away the papers for her, I watched as Milton instantly became calm now that he had a purpose. Diane was patient and caring and took her time in addressing patient needs.

As I walked into my bay, I observed Louise sleeping, Louise had slept for over five hours the longest she had slept in two days. I watched as Louise's mother sat by her bedside stroking her hair as tears rolled down her cheeks.

"Louise works so hard in her job as a dentist, but she rarely takes time for herself, eating the wrong food, not sleeping and drinking heavily. The stroke is a culmination of her unhealthy lifestyle. I hope she will recover," she warned.

"She will," I promised.

"It takes to recover from a stroke, I have supported people in their twenties and thirties who have lived with a stroke before, it can be very traumatic, it takes time to recover emotionally," I replied.

I could feel the tension in the ward. The staff were hot, weak and tired from working from 7 am. Sister Diana had broken the news that a popular night sister called Daisy had died from the virus within a few weeks, whilst other staff across the trust had contracted the virus. There was a feeling of fear in the air from all the other staff. As we walked off the ward at 8pm, a socially distanced crowd outside began to 'clap for the NHS.' We felt so tired and exhausted our faces were covered in marks from the masks, our feet started to hurt, and we were hungry. It felt great to receive so much support from the public, but a part of me felt like we were soldiers putting our lives on the line, with no reassurance from the government that we were being supported.

Chapter 5: The return to the medical ward

Time continued to pass so slowly for all of us, the media appeared to sensationalize the pandemic, showing the surge in people buying toilet roll, and clearing the shelves to prepare for the longevity of the lockdown. During the lockdown, and the initial allowance of going outside twice a day for exercise. I began to observe different types of people. Suddenly I observed joggers wearing luminous brightly colored 80's clothing. I felt like I had entered a time machine. I would then observe several family members going outside for multiple exercise trips, for ice creams, a trip to Tesco's for the fiftieth trip to the park. As each day progressed, I missed my freedom immensely, I missed my trips to the cinema, seeing my friends in restaurants, and going to the gym.

On Saturday the second week of lockdown, I received startling news which shocked me completely. As I awoke to the hot, crisp, sunny morning, I observed my mother had set the table with delicious pancakes, drizzled in the golden syrup and chocolate sauce, and two jugs of orange juice. I looked on in shock at my Mother's expression as she sat looking at the local newspaper.

"Chris, you need to sit down, I have something to show you, please take a seat," she offered.

As I sat at the table, I gasped as I looked at the front cover, I could feel my hands trembling. The picture on the cover was my grown-up childhood friend Charlie, who went missing when he was thirteen. For over two years at secondary school, me and Charlie were inseparable. As my brother Michael hung around with the popular pupils in the football team, I would ride my bike with Charlie to school, and on the weekends we would go on adventures camping in the woods, going to the movies, and setting up a camp in the garden telling each other ghost stories. One day on October 6th, as I attended school, we discovered that Charles had been kidnapped.

Following the weeks after his disappearance, I joined in with the search for Charles. I completed police appeals, we searched the fields with the police, and we reenacted his final steps. I was traumatized by the disappearance of Charles, and I never found as good a friend as Charles in the years after. The news report detailed that Charles was kidnapped by a select religious group, as part of this group he was held for over nineteen years in a boarded-up mansion, with several other children and would spend his time cleaning and completing domestic duties.

At the age of 32, Charles noticed that the front door was open and charged through it running to the police station. After Charles reported the crime he was sent back to the UK and undertook a rehabilitation programmed, which helped him to come to terms with the trauma he endured. The pictures in the paper showed him embracing his mother after not seeing her in nearly twenty years.

"Oh, Chris I think it would be great for you to see Charles, you were both such close friends, you could really help him!" my Mum offered.
"I think I will give him space; I will go and speak to him once he gets used to going home, I think he will need time.

It was so hard to adjust to the news, I believed that Charles had died, I never believed I would find him again, I felt like the year 2020 was filled with so many twists and turns. I felt so anxious each day not knowing what was going to happen next. My parents decided to take Harry to the countryside for the day, on reflection I needed time on my own to comprehend the recent news of Charlie.
I looked at the stack of videos that Michael had recorded that I was lifting on my desk. I decided to watch the videos in short bursts, it made me feel closer to him, I didn't feel alone.

I watched the video, which was recorded around 2009 on our twenty-first birthday. I watched as Michael sat on the sun lounger by the pool in the apartment, sipping on his strawberry milkshake, smiling at the camera, he held his silver twenty-first birthday balloons in his hand.

"Hey Chris, Happy birthday, sorry I can't be with you today. I hope you have the best birthday ever, and I can't wait to see you in the summer. We will have the best time!" he beamed.

I watched as he partied with his friends around the poolside. The outdoor canopy was filled with a range of balloons, party poppers, and a sea of neatly wrapped presents. Meanwhile, I would have been at University in London studying for my acting degree, studying in my room. Whilst my brother was having the best time of his life.

The next shot of the video I observed Michael laying on his couch with head in his hands.

"So, I started my first shift supervising on the ward, and my mentor John complained that we didn't complete the discharges on time. I just feel so tired and weak after the shift, so much is expected of us but there's never enough time!" Michael cried. I watched as Michael looked uncomfortable on the couch, I wondered if the pain could have been a sign that his brain tumor was developing. Michael would complain of headaches regularly the years before he was diagnosed.

The next clip I watched I saw Michael jumping from the cliff from a mountain in the crystal blue sea before the camera faded to black. I felt so close to Michael watching the home movies he created. I wanted to digest the videos slowly. I felt like he was in the room with me.

After I watched the video clips, I received a skype call from my previous flat mate Deborah, who worked alongside me at the local theatre. Deborah was distraught during the phone call, explaining that the theatre was closing, and she was unable to find any temporary work in between. Deborah was distressed after her landlord gave her a final eviction notice for not paying the rent. It was so distressing to see the effect the pandemic had on Deborah, and my fellow actors being unable to find work. Some of my colleagues decided to retrain for other jobs or gained positions in office-based roles in New York City.

After the weekend, and the drama that unfolded regarding my friend Charles, I was ready to return to work and keep busy during the stressful time. I made a conscious effort not to watch the news early in the morning, trying not to increase my anxiety at the time.
It felt like I was back to my previous way of life, rushing my breakfast in the morning, and running to the hospital down the cobbled path hoping to arrive on time. As I arrived at the hospital, I observed various signs all over

the walls, 'stay safe, face, wash hands, and keep 2 meters apart,' and 'no visitors' written on the doors of the wards.

I was happy when I arrived at the Manager's office that I would be working on a general medical ward. As I arrived in the handover room the morning staff looked nervous and tired, hidden behind their visas and white masks. The sister Beth explained that she was dismayed that two members of staff had called in sick with coronavirus symptoms. With the lack of staff on the ward, we were left concerned that we would struggle during the day and require assistance.

I discovered I was working in Bay G, a bay hidden at the corner of the ward in a bay with two patients in the side room, including a man with suspected coronavirus symptoms.

In the first bed was Jack, an eighty-three-year-old man with lung cancer. Jack was struggling to come to terms with his illness following an exacerbation of his symptoms. Jack was a keen sportsman and enjoyed playing football and cricket all his life. I observed Jack sitting in the red recliner chair, despondent, burying his head in his book refusing to acknowledge me.

The second patient was William, a seventy-two-year-old man admitted with an exacerbation in his type one diabetes condition, coinciding with his pre-existing heart failure. I was yet to discover that I had a connection with William that would leave me in shock.

The third patient was eighty-nine-year-old Raymond, a former Jazz singer in the 70's admitted following a report from social services that he was refusing to let carers in, causing him to gain an infection in his leg ulcers. Raymond would sing classic Motown songs on the ward like 'my girl' and Ben E King's stand by me' In a time of fear and worry Raymond was the much-needed positive boost we needed on the ward.

The fourth patient was Samuel, a seventy-nine-year-old man admitted with confusion, and a suspected Urinary tract infection. Samuel was up all night on the ward wandering with his frame, and lay sleeping on his chair, exhausted.

In the side room, one was Lydia, an eighty-year-old woman admitted with a progression in her Alzheimer's condition. Lydia was an ex-nurse and sometimes believed that she was part of the staff team on the ward and required reassurance that she had retired over twenty years ago.

Inside room two was Martin, a ninety-two-year-old man admitted by the community nurse team for end-stage renal care, doctors had confirmed that he was in the final stages of his condition. Martin was a soldier in World war 2 and would discuss with me fascinating stories from his time as a soldier in World War 2.

I worked in the G bay with the healthcare assistant Marie who was quite difficult to work with and would constantly leave the ward to smoke cigarettes.

In the morning Marie and Jane completed the wash and dressing duties together, working to the target of completing the task by 10 am. Suddenly the ward was full of different staff members. The housekeeper zoomed into the ward in her pink dress shouting, "Tea Cake and biscuits anyone." The ward manager Rita ran nervously between bays, asking for updates about our patients and checking the bed states.

The medication round was completed with great difficulty. Jack stated he was too depressed to take his medication, Raymond proceeded to sing the full version of 'Queen, 'the great pretenders' before he consumed his tablets. Whilst Sam stated he wouldn't take my tablets because he feared they may contain poison. Whilst I completed the tasks, I was given several requests from the sister on the ward, 'to chase bloods,' 'ring relatives' and complete bed audits.

I would watch Marie in between her wash and dressing duties running back and forth to the cigarette shelter for a cigarette, I could see the smoke evaporate in her curly hair and the strong smell made me feel sick.

I explained to Jack how I had arranged a meeting for him to discuss the palliative care support he was entitled to receive.

"Look, Chris, I don't want to go into a care facility, I want to just go back to my flat, I don't want to catch the virus, I just want to go home."

"It would benefit you to look into medication and treatment options, we want to make sure that you are pain-free," I explained.

"I don't want to go through chemotherapy treatment, I have been through it before, I don't want to feel tired and weak, but I will talk to the team," He smiled. I watched as Jack reached into his dresser pocket and showed me medals, he achieved in his sporting career and a picture of him with his Manchester football mates. As a nurse, it is important to respect the wishes of patients and to support them to make best interest decisions without influencing our personal beliefs.

After I walked into my bay, I watched as a calmness descended, Raymond was singing, Sam was walking around defiantly with his buzzer asking patients to guide him towards the exit. Martin was sleeping in his bed, whilst Lydia was hoisted into her chair and was watching morning television.

I kneeled beside Raymond to complete the dressings on his ulcerative legs. Raymond started singing, 'stand by me' and encouraged me to sing along.

"No, I won't be afraid, no I won't shed a tear," I smiled. Raymond was a respected singer and travelled all over the country as a jazz artist performing at weddings and funerals. Ever since Raymond's family were involved in a ski accident, he became depressed leading him to reflect his own personal care needs. As I completed the dressing Raymond moved onto singing, 'my girl from the temptations' Suddenly a ninety-year-old lady Shelly from another stood smiling.

"Oh, sir you have a beautiful voice, please can I have this dance?" she asked. I watched as Raymond jumped up and smiled and led Shelly into a waltz in the bay. I watched as the bay of patients sang 'my girl' whilst the other staff congregated to the bay to watch the dance. It was a great moment of escapism from the high-stress levels we were under.

As I walked over to William, I looked into his eyes and observed that he looked so familiar, I felt like I had known him for years, and my curiosity was about to be revealed when I looked inside William's photobook by his bedside. In the photo album was a picture of William as a child standing by an old farmhouse with my Grandfather.

"This photo! I have the same photo at home. This is my Grandfather Richard."

"Well, I am astonished that it would make you my nephew, I'm Richard his brother."

I stood in complete shock and could feel my hands trembling. My Grandfather had spoken of Richard very little, explaining that he had married very young, to a woman who went against his parent's belief and was treated as an outcast by the family. Richard moved to America and studied to be a doctor and lost touch with his family for over fifty years.

"I'm sure you've heard so much about me, your great Grandparents never accepted my wife who was from a very different cultural and religious background, my Father stated if I married Gabrielle, I would no longer be part of the family group."

"That is desperately sad, well I must say it's so wonderful to see you." I smiled.

I watched as Richard began to cry and rested his hand into his head in shock, "Can you just give me a few minutes I just need to process this," he smiled.

I left the room in complete shock, working as a nurse was unpredictable at the best of time, but to meet a long-lost family member completely shocked me. I expected Davina McCall to come onto the ward with her camera!

Marie explained that Raymond's daughter was ringing.

"Hello, I am Michelle, Raymond's daughter. What time is it visiting?" She asked.

"I am sorry, but we are closed for visitors due to the coronavirus."

"Closed? Your hospital ward is open for twenty-four hours!"

"No due to the coronavirus we cannot allow visiting due to the risk of infection"

"Right I'm starting to get very angry! I want to speak to your manager!" she raged.

I passed the phone reluctantly to the sister in charge who repeated the conversation. So many family members were desperate to see their relatives and having to turn them away was heartbreaking. Many of the relatives would ask to see family members in times of crisis.

As I left the phone call, I walked up to G Bay to find my patient Lydia sitting in the bay writing in the patient files. Lydia believed that she was still a nurse and reverted to her younger self.

"Excuse me, can I help you, please? I'm nurse Lydia,"

"Hi Lydia, can you come to the nurse station with me? I want you to help me with a task." I offered.

"No, No, I do not respond to children!" she snapped.

Marie encouraged Lydia to walk towards her room by offering her chocolate cake and a warm cup of tea,

Suddenly I could hear shouting at the front of the desk, it was my patient Sam who had taken another patient's suitcase and was demanding to go home.

"Please I want to go home. I need to return to see my Mum!" he shouted. Senior Sister Kate advised me that I needed to ring the head office to send a health care assistant to provide one to one support to Sam. It was very stressful supporting patients in the ward who were confused or living with dementia. The ward environment was noisy, chaotic and built without structure, which exacerbated the symptoms of the patients.

As I completed the nursing care plans, I attempted to switch off from the staff talking about the virus. In the hospital I felt consumed by it, I wanted to carry on working without discussing it.

I walked into Martin's room, every hour, both myself and Marie would help to turn Martin in the bed in order to prevent pressure sores. In order to prevent the spread of the infection, we had to wear a hospital gown, gloves and a mask under the visa. It made caring for a patient in a hot room very uncomfortable. I was fascinated as I sat beside Martin and he began to recall stories of his time in the army.

Martin explained that he became a soldier at seventeen and joined with his best friend Alan. Martin described the night in battle which changed his life forever. Martin explained that it was a starlit night, he was fast asleep laying his head on his rucksack in the trench. There was not a single sound, for thirty days it rained, and it started to snow. Martin stated it was the first time he had seen snow. In the distance, he could hear a distant voice shouting for help. Martin watched as Alan crept out of the trench holding onto his rifle defiantly. As Martin looked up, he realized it was a trap the soldier crying for helped tricked the soldiers out of the trench.

Suddenly chaos occurred on no man's land, with gunshots flying out, and Martin remembered his heart pounding against his chest with fear until he found a tall oak tree which he hid behind with a fellow soldier Daniel. As they sat cowering behind the tree, just as they were discovered, Alan jumped in front of the bullet saving both Martin and Daniel. Martin explained that he felt too young and too innocent to take on the responsibility of being a soldier, and his life changed forever after his friend passed away. Martin stated that after he exited the army, he went onto become a priest and then studied to be a pharmacologist.

I could have listened to Martin's story all day but due to my nursing responsibilities, I had to meet the needs of all the patients. I helped to provide Martin's medications intravenously, and I assisted him onto the commode, and after I provided personal care, I went to the kitchen to give Martin a warm hot chocolate.

At times as a nurse, I found it hard under the time constraints and envied the carers, who were able to spend more time with patients.

Finally, the healthcare assistant Amelia arrived on the ward and was able to supervise Sam to prevent him from escaping, I finally felt like I could breathe again.

As I walked through the ward, I could hear a silent cry in the visitors' room. I walked in to find Ashley, a first-year student crying as she sat on the couch, Ashley's face was red, and her eyes were puffy.

"What's wrong Ashley?" I asked.

"I'm really struggling, Kate is my mentor, but she keeps expecting too much of me, I've never worked on a ward before, she is constantly testing me, constantly putting me down, criticizing every task!" she cried.

I emphasized with Ashley, having worked with a difficult mentor when I was a student. I offered Ashley the support I wish I had undertaken as a student. I advised her to record negative interactions, try to resolve any disagreement with her mentor in a private meeting. I strongly advised Ashley that if the situation worsened, she would need to inform her ward manager, and the practice placement team, who may be able to provide her with a new mentor.

As I walked to the nurse's station, I met Dr Smith who explained that Bill, my uncle, was about to be discharged and I had to arrange his tablets for going home. I walked over to Bill and passed his medication in a plastic bag as he sat on the hospital chair. Bill grabbed onto my hand as I watched his eyes fill with tears. Bill passed on his childhood photo album, which contained photos of his life with my Grandad when he was a child.

"Listen, I'm so sorry I was not there for you or your family when you were younger, tell your Father I asked for him, I have written a letter to him, in the photo album. I watched as the porter escorted Bill off the ward. I watched in awe, Bill looked so much like my Grandfather, I would never forget meeting him, it felt like a part of history.

Before I finished my shift, I went into the side room to help reposition Martin. I looked on in shock, and I realized Martin had passed away, I checked his pulse and held onto his cold hand. I suddenly felt overwhelmed with emotion looking after a man who served for the country, with such bravery and lived such an interesting life. Martin had so many wonderful stories to tell, and there was so much more I wanted to ask him. I observed how content he was laying in his bed holding onto his rosary beads. I left the room to make the phone call to his daughter to come onto the ward.

"It was an honor to look after you Martin, I hope now you finally find peace," I whispered. I then went over to his cabinet and placed the war medals next to him on his bed. It always reminded me, when each patient that passed away, how fragile life is.

As I looked around the ward, I could see how tired the staff were, we were all under pressure to discharge the patients as soon as possible, as it was the weekend and there was a growing demand for patients to enter the ward. Although Marie had frequently left the ward over a hundred times a day, she worked hard in order to provide the best support to patients. I had struggled through the entire shift on the medical ward, after twelve hours I was tired, hungry and thirsty. I missed my break due to the shortages of staff on the ward and having to take on further responsibilities.

I walked home at half seven, listening to my favorite songs by Elvis Oasis and Keane on my iPod. The ward environment was always stressful and tiring, but I had never experienced the hospital environment being stressful. The pandemic impacted all the staff on each ward and had a huge impact on morale.

I arrived home at 8pm, and observed that Harry was fast asleep, and I sat on the kitchen table with my parents and enjoyed my curry and soft drinks. I broke the news to my parents about meeting William, my Uncle on the ward. I observed the look of shock on my Father's face, he slowly left the room, being unable to speak in shock. My mother warned me that my Father needed time to comprehend the news I had revealed. Then I went upstairs to have a warm bath before collapsing into my warm bed. I lay on top of the single sheet and fell asleep to the sound of a choir of crickets in the background.

Chapter 6: Isolation

I had only been back in England for three months, but I felt like my whole world had been turned upside down. I liked to plan for the future, I wanted to travel the world, visit my relatives in Australia. The pandemic appeared to be taking over the whole world.

A few days after working on the Medical ward, I began to develop symptoms of covid 19, I began to cough constantly, and my temperature was raised. I booked a home test and began the two-week isolation in the loft conversion. It was so hard being away from Harry and my parents for breakfast, lunch and dinner. My parents would leave me a meal at the bottom of the ladder.

I found coping with change very difficult and being stuck in the loft left me feeling more alone. I spent the first few days resting in bed watching my favorite films including 'forrest Gump' and 'the wizard of oz.' I was physically exhausted and weak and would sleep for most of the day. Three days later It was confirmed that I was positive with the virus.

I already felt like I had been in the loft for a month, but I decided I needed to remain positive and not give into my anxious feelings. I stepped off onto the balcony and smiled as the snow silently fell.

In order to cope with being trapped in the loft, I decided to keep busy. I discovered paints hidden in a box and began to paint the walls. As I looked through the stacks of boxes, I discovered a photo album created by my brother Michael. The photo album brought back so many memories from our graduation to our first day at school, and our first trip to Barbados. I realized when my brother passed away that he lived his life to the full for someone in their early twenties. Michael travelled the world, achieved his dream of becoming a doctor and touched the lives of every person that he met. Before he died Michael ensured that messages and gifts were left for me, my sister, and parents to help with his passing.

Throughout the days I felt my cough grow stronger, my fever appeared to erupt during the day. I had now lost my taste and would spend most of my days hidden under a sea of blankets, waiting for the time to pass.

I observed a home video that Michael recorded in the second year of his studies. I realized through watching the video the struggles Michael faced. In the video, he explained he was living with depression and anxiety and was taking Prozac. Michael recorded the home video from his room and explained that he felt so under pressure as a doctor, working under pressure to complete his competencies, and he struggled to adapt to different environments and moving between wards.

I then observed Michael in New York, shopping with his girlfriend, ice skating, and watching a theatre show. Michael encouraged my passion for the city, I enjoyed the sites of the city, the atmosphere, and the friendly nature of people in the town. At the end of the video, I observed Michael's girlfriend holding the camera, and he expressed he was having severe headaches. I wondered why he did not seek help at the time.

I found it difficult communicating with my parents and Harry by phone. I discovered that Harry was still struggling to settle into nursery and expressed how he missed his hometown. For the first week my symptoms worsened as I began to cough more aggressively, I struggled with my appetite, and I began to have very vivid nightmares of being chased by the police.

In my final day in isolation, I felt a creak in the floorboard, as I lifted the floorboard and I discovered a white box, filled with cash, in total 10,000 pounds. After my brother passed, we discovered that the money from his bank account had disappeared, and he had hidden money in the house and garden. I took another test and realized it was negative, I was finally free and was able to have human contact, and I was ready to start work again.

I was so happy to return to work and get into a routine again. Living in isolation, I hated being trapped inside my home and felt like I was a prisoner.

I arrived at the hospital at 7 am and was shocked to discover that I was returning to the Accident and Emergency department. When I arrived at the department I arrived on an unusual day, there were very few patients, and a great team was present. Nurse Josie was a senior nurse with over thirty years of experience as a nurse, my two colleagues Deborah and Lisa were looking after three patients each. Nurse Josie was a magnificent nurse who valued the contribution of all nurses on the ward. At the start of the night shift, Josie brought in a selection of sandwiches and doughnuts for us to enjoy.

I waited apprehensively at the nurse station, waiting for the patients to come in. I helped Julie to complete her admissions. An hour into my shift I received my first patient, Luke, who suffered a minor injury whilst playing rugby. Luke had a big graze on his knee and a temporary bandage on his leg. At sixteen he was one of the youngest patients I had treated. I looked at the fear in his face, as I helped him transfer onto the hospital trolley. Sister Joyce had already contacted Luke's parents.

"It hurts, it stings!" he shouted.

I Prepared a dressing, cleaned the wound before stitching the wound.

"Thank you so much, that feels much better already" Luke exclaimed. I watched as Sister Joyce provided Luke with a cassette player so he could listen to the radio. I then observed Luke's anxious parents rush onto the ward in floods of tears. I always found child nursing difficult and realized how easier it was to support adults.

Two hours into my shift, I was greeted with two admissions at the same time. One patient was George, an ex-convict, admitted after a brawl in a bar, George was accompanied by two policemen and his hands were handcuffed to the hospital chair. George required stitches on his nose, and on his head, which contained pieces of glass from the attack with a wine bottle. George was extremely angry as the police wheeled him in, "What are you looking at you bastard?" he roared. George had long black curly hair, and his face was pure red with rage. The police warned me that George had been released recently for murder. As a nurse, you must accept patients regardless of what they have done and treat them with the care and compassion which was required of us.

Then there was Elaine, an eighty-year-old lady, admitted with confusion and shock after setting fire to her own house. As the paramedics pushed her on the trolley, she held a box of her photo albums which she managed to save from her house. I watched as Elaine began to shake with fear. The doctors crowded around her, assessing her for smoke inhalation. Elaine was covered in black smoke; her white pajamas were black.

After the doctors assessed Elaine, I conducted observations and revealed to Elaine that her observations were in the normal range.

"Oh, I'm so sorry for causing all this trouble, I didn't mean to set fire to the house. I just forget to turn off the cooker sometimes, I struggle with my memory," she explained.

"How often does this happen? Your memory difficulties?" I asked.

"Well my memory has gradually eroded over time, sometimes I wake up to find the front door open, sometimes I find that I've left the fire on when I go out. I've also been having strange visitors in my house, asking for money and sometimes they ask for money." she cried.

I clearly began to see how vulnerable Elaine presented herself to me, leaving the door open and possibly giving money to strangers. I realized I had to complete a referral to social services, a referral and a mental health assessment to support Elaine. As I turned around Elaine was fast asleep, exhausted from the traumatic event that occurred. I covered her in two warm blankets, whilst I waited for the staff on the medical ward to come to assess her.

I then walked up to George, and I was petrified and nervous in inserting stitches into an aggressive patient. As I walked up to his table, I accidentally knocked into his table, causing his jug of water to spill all over the floor.

"Look at you, you're a freak, how can a male be a nurse? You are fucking weird!" he shouted, I watched as his angry brown eyes bore into mine, He was pulling his handcuffs defiantly as he was attached to the bed.

I tried to remain calm, and in my mind, I pictured a scenic beach image as I completed the stitches. George let out a mighty roar as I completed the stitches and frequently called me a bastard through the entire task. As I finished the task, George whispered, "Thank you."

Then in an act of defiance, he spat onto my visa, and I quickly rushed into the sluice to throw away my visa mask and claim another one. In a global pandemic, I was extremely concerned that I could have been exposed to the virus. On the doors of the emergency door were pictures of injured staff, warning patients not to abuse NHS staff, but in my time as a nurse, I was attacked by so many patients.

Sister Josie made me complete an incident report form, and she kindly helped me, by taking over the care of George, as he became more aggressive throughout the shift.

It was then that my next patient arrived, Gillian, a twenty-year-old university student who was admitted following an overdose. Gillian's flat mates found her unconscious in her bed, and when the paramedics arrived, they completed CPR effectively, agreeing that Gillian required one to one support. I watched as Gillian sat crouched on the hospital trolley in her Mr. men pajamas, her eyes filled with tears.

"Please Chris, please don't ring my parents. My Mum will go crazy. I've been depressed for years, and I've just found out that I have failed my second-year medical exams. My parents have been pushing me to join my medical school, like my brother Sean, but I'm finding out it's not the life for me, I want to explore the world, be creative, not stuck in the hospital!" Gillian roared.

I sympathized with Gillian being in the same position myself as a teenager, being pushed to follow my brother's success whilst in reality we were opposites with different dreams.

I completed Gillian's observations observing that they were in the normal ranges and prepared her notes for the assessment ward.

I watched as Julia completed her nursing tasks with ease. I felt like I had not stopped moving all night. Working in Accident and Emergency was an unpredictable environment at best, and required close attention to detail and close assessment skills.

As the night progressed, I was able to steal ten minutes to myself to nibble on my crackers and cheese and drink a few glasses of my sparkling water.

At 5 pm I was exhausted, I could not sit down for very long, fearing I would fall asleep.

As I completed the first morning observations, I could hear a banging at the window. As I looked at the window, I could see a bloodied handprint at the window and a shrill scream. I quickly ran outside through the fire exit and as I looked onto the ground, I observed a twenty-year-old man in a bloodied white shirt holding onto his wound. He had been stabbed in the back, by an empty glass bottle, outside a bar across the road. I quickly removed my nursing Jacket and placed it onto his wound in the first instance before shouting for help. I held the man's head into my hand, and suddenly the staff arrived.

"What's your name?" I asked.

"I'm David,"

"You're going to be ok; we are going to save you. I promised. I helped the nursing staff and doctors rush David into the Emergency treatment room, whilst Josie looked after the patients on my ward. I watched as the doctors worked tirelessly, to close the wound using sulters, while I observed David's heart rate and blood pressure. David was also administered intravenous fluids.

By the end of the shift, I observed David laying on a hospital trolley in the recovery room, and he held onto my hand tightly.

"Chris I want to thank you for helping me, I felt so alone, I thought I was going to die but you were there for me, I wish there was some way I could repay you?"

"No this is my job to care for people, I am so happy that you're going to be ok, I wish you all the best!" I smiled.

I walked home at 7 am to the sounds of the bluebirds tweeting, my legs ached, my feet started to hurt, and I was so tired I could have slept in the field. I arrived into my bedroom at 7:30 am, and collapsed into my bed and began to cry, I was physically drained. I felt during the pandemic I was fighting a battle to save others whilst also fighting to save myself.

I was hoping every day for a vaccine, and for the government to provide more support to the NHS, we needed more staff, PPE equipment, and more guidelines to protect ourselves from the virus.

It was so distressing to hear from my acting friends who were now unemployed, with the widespread closure of theatres and acting projects. I wondered how long it would be until I could return to acting where my heart was.

I celebrated my 32nd Birthday in lockdown when I awoke in the morning the house was filled with balloons, a giant six-tier strawberry cake, and a room filled with an assortment of presents. I received a new laptop, an electronic picture book of times spent with my brother Michael.

As I sat down to the roast dinner prepared by my mother, my Father made a speech.
"Happy birthday Chris, I just want to say we are so thankful that you and Harry are staying with us, and you're not on your own on your birthday. We feel so lucky to have you here, and we know this lockdown has affected your life choices, but we will support you in whatever you do."

At night we gathered around outside and let off our multicolored balloons in memory of Michael. For the first time in three months it felt like events in my life were slowly stabilizing, Harry received a star for good behavior and work at the nursery, whilst I was happy and fortunate to be in a job when so many people were losing their jobs. At the end of my party, I gifted the £10,000 pound I discovered to my shocked parents who had planned to save it for when lockdown ceases.
The following day I received a letter from my old best friend Charlie to meet him socially distanced outside in the town centre. I was excited to see him and discuss what his life has been like and to offer my help so he could move forward. I also received an invitation from my acting agency in New

York, for an online pantomime production of Aladdin. I had so many decisions to make in one of the most difficult times of my life.

Chapter 7: Community panic

I always enjoyed working in community settings as a student and a nurse. Like the hospital, the community setting had an unpredictable nature, from walking into a house with a dog that instantly hates you, to walking into a family reunion. The one element of community nursing that I was particularly fond of was the work/life balance, working 9 to 4 was so much more flexible, in enabling me to have an adequate life/work balance.

I returned to the nurse office and discovered that I was going to be working in the community telephone service centre. The community telephone service consisted of receiving calls from service users, and making outbound calls, to check how patients were coping following discharge. In the afternoon from 1 pm-4 pm, we would visit patients who require a routine checkup. In the mornings if we received an emergency phone call, we would visit the patient immediately to try and resolve the situation.

The telephone office consisted of over forty nurses, answering phone calls, and an on-call physiotherapist and occupational therapist who would often accompany nurses on home visits. As I entered the office I was assigned to work with Celine, a wild flame-haired woman who was very eccentric and sitting next to me was Charity. Charity was very lazy and would often arrive late and would constantly eat snacks at her desk.

As soon as I registered onto the phone, the phone began to ring loudly. I could hear a soft faint cry on the other line.

"Hello, Nurse together line, how can I help you?"

"I'm Richard I was in hospital a few months ago with a UTI infection, now I appear more confused than ever, I am really struggling with my day to day memory, yesterday I forgot my Granddaughter's names I'm so scared." he cried, I could hear the quivering in his voice.

"Do you live on your own, do you have anyone who can support you?"

"No, I live on my own." Richard stammered.

"Would it be ok if we come and visit you this afternoon to have an in-depth conversation and complete our mini mental health test?"

"Yes, that would be great I would be grateful,"

After I hung up the phone started to ring again, it was Doreen, one of the regular callers of the helpline.

"Hi, is that Nurse helpline I am speaking to?"

Hi, It's Chris here, how can I help you?"

"I need to find a word on a crossword here is the clue, it says it is someone related to the world-famous mouse? I mean how can a mouse have a relative or be famous?

"Try Minnie," I smiled.

I could hear Doreen cheering in the background. I then observed Celine hold up a sign which read, 'Tell Doreen we will call her back in the afternoon, ask her if she needs any specific help, Doreen is a regular caller.'

I could then hear Doreen singing as she switched on the radio, singing, "it will be lonely this Christmas without you my dear, you sing now!"

"It will be lonely this Christmas without you Santa," I sang, as the other nurses erupted into laughter.

"Doreen, do you require any help or support today?" I enquired attempting to steer the conversation forward.

"Yes, I need urgent help, I want to raise a safeguarding, my next-door neighbor he is a registered axe murderer and I need help to look for a new accommodation immediately,"

"Ok, I will talk to my manager and see how we can support you," I smiled.

As I hung up the phone call, I discovered that Doreen lived in a mental health facility and was living with schizophrenia and that she rang several helplines a day for help and knew the 'buzzwords' to raise attention or cause for concern. I rang Doreen's warden and she explained that Doreen is perfectly safe, and she lives next to an elderly retired couple who owned the local library.

After the phone call, I paused for a sip of water and a small snack. I observed that everyone in the room was on the phone and busy. It felt great working in a more relaxed environment, without the bright lights, the bleeping of the intravenous machines, and the health workers rushing in and out of the ward.

I observed how bored Charity was as she rested her head into her hands on the desk. "Oh, Chris do you mind making me a hot chocolate, and two digestive biscuits from the kitchen? I'm snowed under," she smiled as she flicked through her magazine. I went to the kitchen to prepare Charity's snack. As Charity took a sip of the tea, she looked on in disgust. "Oh no this is disgusting it has too much sugar in it!" she whined.

Can you make me another one and pick up some letters for me downstairs?" Charity asked.

"Charity just get on with your work Chris is busy."

"I'm busy too, I'm currently snowed under!" Charity whined.

The phone started to ring, "Hi I'm Shirley I just wanted to speak to someone really. I was discharged from the hospital two months ago. I had a fall at home after my husband passed away, and I just feel so alone. I have no one to speak to. I just feel so alone, so depressed, especially during the pandemic, I miss going to my friends. I feel so isolated."

"I understand it must be so hard for you Shirley, but you always have us to speak to and there are a range of online support groups we offer,"

"Support groups would be so helpful, I just don't want to feel alone anymore," Shirley agreed.

It was devastating to see the effect of the pandemic on the elderly in society. With so many services closed and with tight social distancing restrictions so many people felt a deep sense of loneliness. The nursing support line was a lifeline for people who did not have anyone to talk to.

I then received a phone call from a man mistaking the nursing helpline for a Chinese takeaway.

The final phone call was a highly charged emotional call.

"Hi, my name is Maria, I have a huge emergency. My life is in danger!" she panicked.

"Maria, we are here to help you, what is wrong?"

"I can't get up from the toilet. I'm frightened, please help me. I'm on Clifton road."

"We will help you, Maria," I promised.

I spoke to Celine and she explained that Maria was known to the service but had never rung in an emergency, and she only lived five minutes from the nursing office.

We drove to Celine's house just before 12, with Alan the physiotherapist. As we arrived at the house we looked on in complete shock. There were two ambulance trucks outside and a fire engine. We looked at the annoyed expression of the ambulance staff. As we walked into Maria's house, we observed her laying in her duvet on the sofa and a cup of tea.
"Oh, Maria and co, great to see you, no need to worry, two firemen helped me up and now I'm fine.

"Marie if ever you need help in the future and it's not a life-threatening emergency you can call us!"
We stayed and supported Alan in supporting her with mobilizing. The nursing line was often filled with calls from people who called us with 'emergency calls' because they could not access immediate carer support.

We then went to visit George, the man who rang the helpline earlier in the day stating he was living with memory difficulties. We arrived at George's house at 3 pm, he greeted us wearing his red-checkered pajamas and holding his Labrador. All around his house were unopened letters, and a huge mattress was in the dining room covered in packets of crisps and tins of beans. George was very tearful, as we sat down at the small kitchen table.

"I'm so glad you've come to see me, I'm really struggling every day, my memory is so poor I'm worried about my own safety," George stammered. "We are here to help you, is it ok if we complete our mini mental health assessment, just to assess your memory further?"

The mini-mental consisted of questions including memory recall, naming animals, drawing a clock face, and completing mental arithmetic. In order to pass the test, the mark needed was 23/26. George struggled throughout the entire test, only achieving an actual score of ten, which showed a clear deficit in his memory. Alan then assessed George's mobility, noting that he had an unsteady gait, and he struggled to walk upstairs which showed how his mobility was gradually declining. At the end of our visit, we referred Mike to the memory clinic, for further assessment, and he appeared grateful that he was receiving help.

I enjoyed my shift in the community, it was nice not to have the pandemic controlling every aspect of our work. In the hospital, we were constantly washing our hands, surrounded by posters of how to prevent the virus and there was a sense of fear all around us. In the office in the community whilst we were socially distanced, the environment was much more relaxed.

It was wonderful to return home at 5pm, I was able to pick Harry up from Nursery, and we picked up a Wagamama's curry and returned home to an evening of Karaoke and watching our favorite film Edward Scissorhands.
"When can we go home?" Harry asked.
"We will have to wait until this bad bug has disappeared," I promised. In truth I did not know when I would return to the US, there was not much left for me there, and I needed at least I had a sense of purpose during the pandemic.

That evening, I went upstairs and watched another instalment of my brother's home movie. I watched our sightseeing trip on our twenty-first birthday. I travelled to see Michael after a year of being separated, and I observed how different we were. I lived an average life of studying as an actor and working in a bar at the weekends whilst Michael worked as a doctor on the frontline and held lavish parties in his apartment every week with over a hundred of his college friends.

I watched the video of our birthday, as we drove in his Mercedes car towards the Grand Canyon. We had the windows down, and the personalized cd filled with our favorite songs from oasis the Beatles and Elvis. I rested my head back on the seat as the sun scorned my face, I felt so free. We spoke about our hopes and wishes for the future, we planned to open up our own clothes shop, travel the world, and eventually move onto our Grandad's home next to the beach in Alnwick. We arrived at the Grand Canyon at 1 pm, and I was petrified as we climbed up the mountain, although we were harnessed in, I held onto a deep fear that the rope could tear apart. Over an hour later we arrived at the top of the mountain, we shouted at our names and marveled at the view. We observed the doves swooping past us, the dusky mountains looked breathtaking from the top. We then proceeded to cover the beach, a beautiful scenic beach with crystal blue waters. We took it in turns to jump from the mountain top, my heart raced against my chest and I crashed into the ice-cold sea. It was wonderful spending time with my brother, I had the best day in over a year.

We returned later to Michael's luxury apartment, in which his girlfriend Kate had arranged for us. The apartment was filled with hundreds of 21st birthday silver balloons, dancers on stilts, a DJ playing our favorite pop songs, and hundreds of his colleagues at the hospital joined us. We danced all night, everyone sang together, and we enjoyed being twenty-one and looking to the future without knowing how our lives were soon to be changed forever. Watching the home movies Michael created, opened all the feelings of grief I once had.

The following day I was apprehensive, as I had arranged a meeting to visit my childhood friend Charlie. I was so apprehensive and nervous in meeting him but wanted to try my best to help orientate him back to a normal way of life. I decided to bring a scrapbook of old photos of us on the adventures we went on and wanted to share with Charlie all the newspaper clippings I kept since he disappeared.

Over the years following his disappearance, there were many theories about the disappearance. Many people believed he could have been killed by the local town murderer, who was found to have killed over five children in the neighborhood over twenty years. On the internet on certain blog sites, people had reported having seen him in restaurants, theme parks and in the movie theatre.

I took our dog Rex, to the meeting to try and regain a normal feel to the meeting. I arrived at the field at 11 am, and observed Charlie sitting awkwardly on the bench in the cornfield. It was so strange for me to see him as a grown 32-year-old man, I always envisioned him as the eternal twelve-year-old. I looked on in shock at his gaunt expression, his face was so pale, his expression was gaunt, and his hair was long and black. For twenty years, he had not been exposed to sunlight and was trapped inside his captor's house completing chores each day.

"It is so great to see you again Charlie, I never thought this day has come, I can't believe it's been twenty years!"

"I remember the times we had all the bike rides and sitting around the fire at night. Tell me about what life is like for you now? Do you still listen to Oasis? Do you still go on your bike ride?"

I sat and spoke to Charlie for over an hour, he seemed so childlike, he had missed out on so many milestones in life, going to university, getting his first job, going on a date. Every question that Charlie asked related to when he was twelve years old.

I listened in awe at Charlie's devastating story, on the day he was captured he was forcefully pushed into the kidnapper's van. He spent twenty years in the basement of Eric's house with the other children washing linen, cleaning the floors, filing papers. Each day they would drink two bowls of soup and one glass of water. Charlie spoke of the terrible conditions he lived in, sleeping on the muddy floors, surrounded by rats, they were so uncomfortable and would spend most of the night shivering on the stone-cold floor.

Charlie explained that every day felt like Groundhog Day, they felt like slaves working day and night as slaves. Charlie recalled the day he escaped his chapters house, Ethan the main chapter had accidentally left the front door open, Charlie charged towards him hitting him across the head with a clock radio successfully escaping.

We spent the day walking in the field, talking about our high school peers and their current destination. Charles was shocked to hear of my brother's passing and was upset that he had missed out on so much of his life and wished that he could turn back time and start again.

Chapter 8: Community terror

The following day, I arrived back at the nurse's managers office, and was again located on the nursing community team. I was happy to get a break from the manic nature of the covid wards. I was about to spend my shift with the healthcare assistant Lucy. Lucy drove a polo car and would constantly smoke cigars in the car, which meant being in the car with her was incredibly uncomfortable. We had a list of over seven patients to see, including five patients who required nursing care and two patients who required help with personal care.

As I sat in the passenger seat of Lucy's car, I felt uncomfortable as I held onto the seats as she blasted out the greatest hits of Queen in her car. I always found it difficult sharing a car with other care practitioners, adapting to their behavior.

The first patient we visited was Agatha, a ninety-two-year-old lady who required patient education regarding her recent type two diabetes condition. We knocked on Agatha's door for over five minutes.

"It is so unusual Agatha is usually at the door, ready to greet us with a cup of tea." As Lucy peered through the gap in the front door, she observed Agatha laying on the floor. We grabbed the key from the key safe and entered through the back door. As we walked in Agatha was laying beside the front door, in her purple nightgown holding her telephone. As we turned Agatha over, we checked to see her level of consciousness, and as we felt her pulse and freezing cold hands, we realized that Agatha had passed away. We called the ambulance after noting Agatha's 'do not resuscitate' document left on her kitchen dresser. As the ambulance came to take Agatha to the county hospital, Lucy broke down in tears in the car.

"I have looked after Agatha for over fifteen years, she often spoke of the incredible back pain she suffered from ever since she had a major accident in her car. I think she just couldn't cope anymore."

We later discovered that Agatha had taken an overdose of paracetamol tablets, after complaining about the unbearable pain she was in. It was one of the most difficult aspects of nursing, not knowing what situation you were walking to and supporting patients in life and in death.

We then made our way to John Sampson's house, a sixty-five-year-old man who required dressings on his ulcerative legs. John was over twenty stone and lived with his two Alsatian dogs. As we walked into the dining room, we observed John sitting on his rocking chair watching the countdown. In the corner of each room were his Alsatian dogs looking at me in contempt. I could feel my heart racing against my chest as the dogs stared at me, I felt like I was dinner.

Lucy helped me to lift John's legs so I could begin the dressings.

"The dogs will be ok with you, just as long as you don't make any sudden movements," John smiled.

John continued to watch the countdown, shouting out clues to the show. As I wrapped his leg in the honey dressing, I could feel Lucy's hand pressed against my shoulder. "Stay very still, don't move," Lucy warned.

Suddenly John's Alsatian started to bark aggressively, immediately I jumped back in a state of terror, John shouted heel and the dog instantly stopped barking. I was always fearful of going to the houses of clients of people who had animals. As a student, and as a nurse in the community, I encountered so many animals and creatures from snakes to lizards to offensive parrots.

As we drove up the country roads, I struggled to breathe under the thick cloudy smoke from Lucy's cigars. I was shocked to hear that Lucy was reluctant to train to be a nurse due to nurse training not being paid and her ward department refused to train her through work.

I then went to visit our third patient's house, Anita, at 99 she lived alone in a Grande three-story Edwardian mansion and a ten-acre beautiful garden with a badminton court. Our appointment with Anita today was to check on her progress following her fall on her basement stairs.

When we arrived at the house, we looked on in awe at Anita's amazing abilities for her age. As we walked into the dining room Anita proceeded to show us her yoga techniques, in her dance hall. Anita explained that she keeps fir every day by playing Yoga, jogging in the garden, playing badminton with her sister, and running on her treadmill. It was inspiring to see how active Anita was, having lived her life as a dance teacher for over sixty years, she danced every day, ran her own internet blog based on healthy eating, and held lavish parties with the friends she had made over the years.

Anita encouraged us to look at the photos on her wall of all her achievements, her dancing awards, her three-degree certificates, and her PhD certificate. It was so great to meet someone who defied the stereotype of a person of her age.

We then travelled to the next patient's house seventy-nine-year-old Andrew's house. Andrew had previously been admitted to hospital with depression, and our visit to John was based upon reviewing his heart failure medication. I looked after John before on a medical ward previously.

John lived with his wife Imelda. Both John and Imelda were very eccentric, they would argue over the slightest matter, they would sing together and would dance on the ward.

We knocked on the door and Imelda was excited as she opened the door.

"Come in you too, we have prepared a banquet," she smiled.

"Oh, Imelda we can only stay for a half an hour you see-"

"Oh, nonsense! It's John's birthday today and you too are our guests!" she smiled. Imelda took me by the hand into the dining room, to show me the party table, which was filled with a range of sandwiches, multicolored cakes and a three-tier birthday cake. I had to insist with Imelda that we needed to see John as time was pressing. To my Shock Imelda turned on the radio and led me into a waltz into the dining room, singing along to the song, 'time of our lives.' As we walked into the back-dining room, John was resting on the sofa, and the room was filled with hundreds of balloons and confetti.

The house was very unkempt covered in unopened letters, chocolate wrappers and half-opened pizza boxes. We noticed that John had his tablets mixed together in a glass cup.

"Oh John, it might be more beneficial for you to use a blister pack so that you can access your medication more easily. It is very unsafe to mix your medication together; it can have a detrimental effect on your help. I will order you blister packs from now on.

How have you been coping since you were discharged from the hospital? I know you struggled, stating that you found it hard to leave the house and you felt quite lonely?"

"I just feel depressed with my heart failure condition affecting my breathing, and my mobility is affecting me," he cried.

"Well, we have a list of local groups that you could go to, including a history group and exercise class and a cookery group."

Suddenly Imelda burst into a flood of tears as she stood by the curtain and began to pull them off the hook angrily.

"John, I have tried to encourage you to go shopping with me, you won't even join me for a walk in the park. You're not depressed, you're just an absolutely lazy bastard!" she shouted, as she cried hysterically.

Lucy walked over to Imelda, and held onto her trembling hands, in an attempt to calm her down. We were happy that John was compliant in his medication routine and agreed to participate in local groups. As we were about to leave to our shock, Imelda offered for myself and Lucy to close our eyes as they had a surprise for us, they started to countdown from three.

Suddenly Imelda and John popped the confetti cannon covering us in multicolored confetti.

Our Final house on our visit was Mary Andrew, Mary was diagnosed with vascular dementia, and was living on her own in her home. It had been over two months since she was diagnosed, and we were visiting her to check how she was coping and if she required anymore support.
We arrived at Mary's house at 3 pm, she walked towards us in her daffodil dress, struggling with her walking stick.

We walked into the kitchen and noticed all of the Elvis memorabilia she had all over the house. On the walls, she had signed Elvis Vinyl framed on the wall. In the kitchen, she had an Elvis tablecloth on her kitchen table, with an Elvis cup, Elvis cutlery and hundreds of Elvis magnets she collected over the years. We began to see signs that Mary was struggling, in her fridge, many of the items were out of date, she struggled to make a sandwich when prompted, and all her worn clothes were placed in a pile in the kitchen.
"How have you been coping Mary since your discharge from hospital?"
"I prefer to be at home, my neighbors help me with wash and dressing tasks, and my Friend Dolly visits once a week," Mary explained.
Would it be ok Mary if we can organize for an admiral nurse to visit you?

An admiral nurse is a specialist dementia nurse who can help you in looking at managing taking your tablets, they can help you look for carers, and answer any questions you have related to dementia."

Mary then proceeded to talk about Elvis and expressed that she spent all of her first year's wages on a ticket to see Elvis in Las Vegas and explained how she fainted when he touched her hand.

I returned to the district nursing office at 9 am the next day. It was such a hot day I sat with three mini fans hoping I would be able to cool myself down. I sat next to Celine who sat with her nursing notes carefully stacked in a neat pile, as she started to make phone calls. I observed how anxious the nurses were, as they began to handle the distressing calls from the previous patients. Even though the lockdown rules had been eased, schools were opened, and people were returning to work, the effects of the pandemic were echoed in the distressed calls.

Our first call was Ben Thomas, Ben was discharged a month ago after his heart transplant admission.

"Hello Ben, I'm just ringing to check how you are doing following your discharge from hospital?

"Well, I am very concerned the care home manager of my wife's home won't let us visit her. I understand they have had a previous case but it'd been three months. The care home manager has banned visit completely, what should I do? He asked.

"Well Ben each care home has to follow the government guidelines, but you can always check with your local council to check the rules for care homes in your area. You also mentioned that you feel that the care home is having a detrimental effect on your wife's condition, It may be worth writing to your local MP to make them aware of your current situation."

"I have spoken to Jill on the phone and she thinks I am her brother. She cannot recall the marriage at all as her condition has progressed. When this is over, I am going to sue and go to the papers!" he shouted.

I really sympathize with Ben throughout the call; he was clearly very distressed and trying to adapt to the government rules. It was so difficult to offer advice when the government kept changing rules, and we were apprehensively waiting for news on the production of a vaccine.

I discussed with Celine the wide range of calls the staff were facing ranging from patients who were waiting for appointments, delays in cancer treatments, care agencies abandoning services out of the blue. The consensus was that so many patients were in crisis, yet the virus cases were still raised.

The next caller was Tommy, an eighty-nine-year-old man, admitted to a ward two month previously with complications in his diabetes condition. "Hello Nursing together I need help, I'm feeling sick and tired all the time and my cat has gone missing, can you help?"

"Well Tommy I can help discuss with you later today how we can support you by visiting you this afternoon, I can help you look for the cat but I may be pushed for time," I replied. It was always difficult visiting patients of animals. It was terrifying when animals were aggressive, but to find a missing animal made it harder.

The next caller was seventy-one-year-old Sheila, Sheila was put on continuous oxygen, but it limited her mobility, and she requested portable oxygen so that she could see her family outside.
"I just feel so alone, it's been three months since I've seen my family members, and I am just sick of talking to them on the phone. I just want to see them physically. I run my own shopping channel on Instagram, so I am very busy." she smiled.

"I can come and see you this afternoon and we can certainly talk about your options," I smiled. I began to see how isolated the elderly community felt constrained by the lockdown.

I then received a phone call from a lady called Betty, Betty was crying hysterically on the phone and was asking for help regarding her mother who is living with dementia.

"Hi nurse, I'm a teacher on my lunch break but I just need urgent help."

"Sure, how can I help you?"

"Ever since the lockdown my mother is not responding or interacting, she just sits and stares, I'm so concerned? Any advice?

"Is she stimulated? Does she complete any activities?" I asked.

"No Nurse, before lockdown she went to a cafe every day, a thirty-minute walk and a Zumba dance class. Now that the lockdown is here her routine has dissolved."

"Well you could try a number of activities at home to support music therapy has been known to provide stimulation. Reminiscence therapy has shown to support people who are living with dementia, it may be worth getting together old photo albums, or creating a photo album to help your mother look back at past events."

"Well I'm sure I can try, can you come around today?

"Yes, I can come at 4 pm," I replied.

After the call, I drank my cup of tea and watched as Nurse Heather was crying in the corner of the room. Celine was supporting her as she had just returned from maternity leave and was struggling with the drastic changes in her role, moving from calm district nurse visits to constant crisis calls. The final call was from Miles, Miles expressed that he needed help with his mobility as he was struggling following his fall. I arranged to meet Alan the physiotherapist at 3 pm.

In the afternoon I drove along the country roads on my own, I had only been driving for two months and felt nervous. Then disaster struck as I took a wrong turn. I was met by a herd of sheep, I pulled the window down, and shouted for the farmer to move them. As I stepped out of the car, I slipped onto the floor falling into the cow poo. I wanted to run home, so I called Alan to bring a spare uniform and was thankful that I had spare clothes in the boot for the meantime.

I managed to arrive at Tommy's house at 4 pm that morning, I knocked on the door and discovered Tommy running down the corridor, opening the door in panic.
"Oh nurse, I'm so glad you're here. Tiddles my cat in the orange tree. I need your help," he cried. My heart started to pound against my chest, I had participated in cardiac arrests and emergencies but saving a cat

terrified me. As I ran into the garden, I observed the grey kitten stuck on a branch, whilst the step ladders were placed next to the tree.

"I can't reach him, and I don't want the RSPCA involved.

I took a deep breath, and I climbed up on the ladder and managed to pick up the shivering kitten, placing it in Tommy's hands. Thomas shook my hand repeatedly, thanking me for my kindness.

Tommy then guided me towards his fridge, I noticed the unhealthy foods he was eating. In the fridge were several pizzas, three chocolate cakes, three crates of sugary drinks and ice cream boxes. I realized how the food would have a strong impact on his diabetes condition.

As we sat on the couch, we discussed limiting the fats and sugar in his diet and subsisting the healthy foods with healthy portions of carbohydrates and proteins.

It was then that Tommy broke down in tears, "I just feel so alone since my wife and kids left me, food is a comfort to me you see, it helps me when I feel low," he smiled.

"Well you can talk to us, we are always here for you, and we can book you in to speak to your GP to discuss talking therapy, it may make you feel more positive. Exercise can be helpful too, we can offer many support groups," I explained. I offered a range of booklets to guide Tommy.

"Thank you for your help, it really helps to talk to people, it is wonderful to have a nurse that understands." he smiled.

I then went to visit Sheila and as I knocked on the door she peered around the corner of the door. "Sorry, Chris I'm really busy. I have a deadline for an order for tomorrow. Come tomorrow!" she smiled. It was not uncommon for patients not to accept a visit, I once heard a patient shout "Tell that flaming nurse I'm not in," whilst I was knocking on the door.

I then reached Betty's house where she lived with her mother Lucy. When I pulled up Betty looked on in happiness and excitement, "oh nurse come in, you will not believe it," she smiled. I walked into the dining room to observe Lucy sitting on her rocking chair smiling and laughing, as she looked through images of her childhood, her wedding day, and holiday photos.

"Mum has really responded to the photographs; I can't thank you enough. Even the CD player has helped to alleviate her mood. When my mother was diagnosed, I was just given the diagnosis by the doctor and left to it, but you have really helped to explain things. Thank you!" she beamed.

I then went to meet Andy the physiotherapist at Miles house. Andy laughed as he heard about my incident at the country road. We then went to visit Miles. Miles opened the door and to our surprise, he was joined by his identical twin brother Harry. They were both wearing matching yellow dungarees. "Hi welcome to our home," they smiled in unison. I felt like I had just stepped into the house of a famous duo. As I looked on the walls, I saw photos of the twins with famous quiz show contestants such as Noel Edmonds and Barry White. "We have been on over fifty gameshows in our lifetime. We are the Davies twins, surely you recognize us?" he smiled. We saved up our money and started up our own travelling circus which we have run for over thirty years."

"Wow, that is amazing really," I smiled trying to observe the flood of information. The entire house was decorated with clown memorabilia, and circus pictures were imprinted on the floors.

I assisted Alan to help to assess Miles mobility, and Andy assessed that he no longer needed a new walking stick and instead required specialist footwear. Before we let Miles and his brother offer to put on a magic show for us, but we had to be back by the office for 3:30 pm. A part of us felt like the twins just wanted company, like many of the others we had seen but due to time constraints, we had to move on.

When I returned home that evening, I looked on in shock, as I entered the room, I observed Six puppies running around the house. It was a chaotic scene, one puppy was chewing on new trainers, whilst another puppy had destroyed the frames of my designer sunglasses. Harry was in heaven running after the puppies.

"Mum, what is going on?" I asked

"Well this morning it was revealed that I will be losing my job, I really needed to cheer myself up, so I bought the puppies." she smiled. Mum had worked in the library for over thirty years, it was devastating to see the effects of the pandemic.

That evening Charlie arrived at the house, and as he stood on the doorstep, he proceeded to update me on his current situation.

"Thank you, Chris, for talking to me, so much has happened since I lost sight of you. It has been revealed that Eric and the other captors have been given life in prison. I have just gained a position as a Checkout worker at John Lewis and I have enrolled into college to complete my G.C.S.E's."

"Wow Charlie, it seems your life is really coming together, you're doing really well!"

"Well I have to keep busy, I've missed out on twenty years of my life, and I need to start rebuilding my life, I refuse to sit at home and contemplate on what's happened," he smiled. I admired Charlie for his courage in trying to improve his life. Each day and each week of the pandemic came with so many changes. I lived by a routine and now felt like I was living in a film without a script.

I enjoyed spending time in the community setting, but I know I would only be in the community for a limited time. With the rise in covid cases and the need for staffing on the wards, I knew I would be needed on the ward.

The following day I returned home that afternoon and observed how upset my parents were after crashing their BMW into a parked car. It was then that they ushered me to sit at the kitchen table, I knew it was going to be a serious conversation.

"We've both been thinking lately about the future, and we have decided we want to sell the house, it's just too big for us now and we want to be closer to you and Harry. We want to move to New York."

"You can't leave here, it's our childhood home, it holds so many memories for all of us, what about Michael's belongings?" I cried. I was thinking selfishly of myself thinking that selling the home would erase the final traces we had left of Michael.

"We will rent a cottage in Yorkshire and you and Harry are welcome to stay whilst the pandemic eases. We just feel now is the time for us all to move on with our lives, and a big part of this, will be moving from this house." she smiled.

I went upstairs that evening and watched the final video Michael had made. It showed Michael aged twenty-four, the year he was diagnosed with cancer. Michael made the video following his office room in a GP surgery in Yorkshire. Michael was happy that he finally passed his finals, and that his ambition now was to become a registered GP practitioner. Michael explained that he had now made one hundred thousand pounds in total in his freelance clothing company.

Everything now started to become clearer, after Michael's passing, he had left money for me and our other family members, which he kept hidden in boxes, often leaving clues for us to find it. That night as I lay in bed, I knew it was the right decision for my parents to move to a new house, and it would be the final step needed for me to move forward to the future.

Chapter 9: The battle continues

I arrived the next day at the nurse Manager's office, ready to take on my next challenge. I was placed in the Accident and Emergency ward on a very manic day. As I stepped onto the ward, I witnessed chaos and hysteria. Three paramedics appeared with three people who were involved in a major RTA, the night nurses were ready in the treatment room with the doctors to assess them. Suddenly an elderly couple dressed in mink coats stormed towards the senior sister on the ward, demanding a covid test despite the signs and public announcements not to attend the emergency services for tests. The night nurse and senior nurse were busy in the bedroom, attending to a patient who had fallen in the bedroom, meaning that our handover was delayed.

I was then introduced to my bay of patients from cubicle B to G. The first patient was Emily, an eighteen-year-old girl who accidentally fell from her balcony at a university party. Emily's leg was placed in the caster. The second patient was John, a 55-year-old builder, admitted following having a heart attack following his unhealthy daily habits.
Martha was 90, a cheery lady who was admitted with a chest infection and was recovering from a minor fall in her house.

In bed E was a lively eighty-five-year-old man admitted following a fall from a flight of stairs at home, and it was suspected that he had broken his ankle.

The final patient in bay G was Emily a twenty-eight-year-old nurse, admitted following an attempted suicide attempt, following the breakup of her boyfriend.

Today I was working alongside a newly qualified nurse Rebecca, who had only worked on the ward for a week and required support.

I completed the medication round with ease, but I had to convince Clive that his blood pressure tablets were necessary to support him as he suspected he was being poisoned.

Suddenly I could hear Martha screaming out from the side room. I walked in to find Martha looking angry and concerned. "What is all that noise out there? She asked.

"It is just really busy out there this morning," I exclaimed.

"Well tell them to keep it down," she smiled. I encouraged Martha to use her nebulizer as she became breathless. I observed with fascination at Martha's creations on her bed, on her two days of admission she had knitted over fifty baby cardigans, despite being desperately ill.

Unlike the community environment, in which I had time to reflect and rest in between patient visits, I always had to be alert. Clive was very confused and tearful and required constant reassurance of his whereabouts. I had to be stern with John who proceeded to walk around the ward and help himself to coffee despite suffering from a major heart attack.

"John you must sit down, you need to rest, you must not exert yourself as you have been such a traumatic event. "

"Listen Chris I've got jumpers older than you. I think I know at 55 how to care for myself. I just wish I did not let life events get to me, you see my seventeen-year-old daughter has just revealed she is pregnant, my son is recovering after spending time in rehab for drug addiction. Then we have been hit by a pandemic!" he groaned.

I had noticed that so many patients had been affected by the pandemic. I discussed with John a healthy diet plan and explained that he would need to spend time on the cardiac ward to be monitored, much to his anger.

I had observed throughout the shift how Emily's mood seemed to deteriorate as time went by. I observed her crying on her bed with the curtain drawn to hide her grief.

"Emily the ward psychologist Beth is due on the ward in an hour and she will want to see you," I assured her.

"I'm not sure what good that will do. My boyfriend Jake has split up with me, we were together for two years, I've lost my home, my job and my friends all in one month. I just can't cope!"

"I'll be here if you need me," I offered

I then went to help turn Sara who was about to be transferred to a medical ward, Sara was optimistic following her fall, but was fearful of breaking university rules for partying and was wary of the consequences.

I was so busy during the shift and so consumed by paperwork that I managed to miss my first break. I was always pushing myself to take breaks, to support my own personal wellbeing as not having breaks makes me feel weaker and tired.

During the shift, I witnessed that the NQN nurse Rebecca became increasingly stressed and sat crying in the medication room. I observed her sloped on the floor in desperation.

"What's wrong Rebecca? You have been doing a great job."

"I'm just so stressed, I have been in the ward for over a month and I've got so much to learn like cannulation, taking bloods, and setting up Iv's. I'm just so stressed with the pandemic, I have to isolate myself from my friends and my parents are in the vulnerable category," she sobbed, as I passed her tissues.

"Rebecca being an NQT nurse is a learning process, you will have your good and bad days, but remember you can only achieve your competencies with the support of others, ask me if you need any support," I assured her.

As I returned to the ward, that afternoon, I experienced a relaxing end to my shift, Clive and John were sent to medical wards for further assessment, whilst Sara was sent to a recovery orthopedic ward. Emily felt more settled after speaking to the psychologist, whilst Martha had made twenty more cardigans.

I returned home to a shock, my parents had taken Harry to dinner, and I could hear crying in the spare room. I was petrified as I did not expect anyone to be in the house. As I crept up the stairs, I observed my sister Louise crying on the double bed. My sister had been estranged from the family for two years due to a family argument.

"Louise, what's wrong? I have not seen you in so long.

"It's Mike, he left a note on the stairs, this morning, he's finally left, the marriage is over" She sighed.

"I'm so sorry Louise, have you tried to call him? Where are the kids?" I asked.

"We are staying at my friend Dawn's house, but you don't understand I'm so happy he has left. Mike is the reason I don't see you or Mum and Dad, he has become more and more controlling, he has locked us in during the pandemic, he has hit me several times. Now I am free, I'm crying because I'm relieved," She smiled.

I listened in shock. My sister's husband was always presented as a kind, gentle person and like many couples, during lockdown, they struggled immensely under the pressure, and Louise succumbed to domestic abuse.

I then observed Louise get up and run down the stairs towards the door.

"Where are you going?" I shouted.

"Chris please don't tell Mum and Dad I was here. I just need time to get my life together," she cried.

I looked on in shock, as Louise drove off into the distance.

Chapter 10: Winter pressure

I arrived at the winter pressure ward which was specifically opened to look after patients with various medical illnesses. Staff were regularly tested for covid, and if patients were showing symptoms of the coronavirus, they were isolated in one of the ten side rooms. I was working alongside Hayley, one of the most patronizing nurses' I had ever worked with. Hayley would call me Tony and would talk to other staff below her pay grade in a squeaky voice. The other sister, Jenny, was a much-loved nurse, who would always help staff and would sing throughout the shift.

I was supporting patients with a range of medical needs. In the side room I supported Amelia who was living with worsening symptoms of her MS, her mother was with her, and would constantly ask questions.

In the bay was Thomas, an eighty-nine-year-old man living with advanced dementia. Thomas was a toolmaker and had a range of materials to help make items such as toy wooden cars. Tommy was admitted due to not complying with his carers, and required a future assessment of his condition.

Then there was 90-year-old Mick, Mick was admitted after having palpitations, after previously having open-heart surgery. Mick would constantly press the buzzer, just to have a conversation with staff members.

Then in the sixth bed was Claude, a 100-year-old previous consultant, he was living with terminal cancer. Around his bedside were flowers, plants, and hundreds of cards from his friends and ex-colleagues. Today he was receiving a visit from his Labrador retriever Tabby, as a special request due to the worsening of his condition.

The final patient was Gill in the side room, Gill was admitted with confusion, and was a previous OFSTED inspector and would move rapidly with her Zimmer frame, 'inspecting' workers.

I really struggled in the morning, as two healthcare assistants called in sick, and I had to complete the washing and dressing tasks on my own. Already, I felt so stressed, but Jackie the senior sister stepped in to help with the washes, saving me from going on fire!

I was then called into the side room, as Amelia's mother had some concerns about her daughter. "When is Amelia going to be discharged? Why have we been waiting for a consultant? Who can I complain to about her treatment?" she roared. I tried to answer her questions explaining that the consultants do not usually work at the weekend.

"Go on move along, you are talking like a politician at the moment avoiding questions!" she roared.

I then observed Gill charging through the ward along the corridor, with her Zimmer frame, at moments she would stop and observe the staff in each B.
"Gill would you like to take a seat, and have a cup of tea? You have been walking all morning." I offered.
"No, I'm far too busy. I have to inspect St Helen's Primary school at 11 pm" she warned. I then found a folder and a notepad for Gill. Gill sat down and recorded her observations, believing she was assessing teacher performance. Whilst Gill had a purpose in writing her notes and was stimulated, she began to drink more and enjoyed her snacks.
I then observed Hayley sitting at the desk, barking orders. When I walked around the nurse's station, I observed Hayley wearing an assortment of doughnuts and playing Tetris on her phone.
"I do hope you complete some discharges today Tony," She barked.

I then observed Claude's daughter arrive with his Labrador retriever. Claude had been feeling quite depressed in his bed and had refused to engage with family and staff for a week. As soon as the Labrador entered the closed curtains, he jumped onto the bed next to Claude. I watched as Claude smiled and tears fell from his eyes, knowing that it may be his final encounter with his pet. I watched as the Labrador rested its head on Claude's shoulder, and calmly fell asleep next to him, as Clade began to stroke his head. It was wonderful that the hospital allowed Claude to spend time with his pet.

I was then called by the wife of Thomas; she was distressed as Thomas was in the bathroom but was refusing to wash.

"I don't know why Chris, but he simply refuses to wash any tips."

"It may be worth giving him a purpose to wash by saying after you wash, we can go for a walk. You could also try bringing in new pajamas or fragrant body wash to help encourage him." I offered.

"I will try to thank Chris," she smiled. I later discovered that Thomas was reluctant to go to the shower after having a fall and would only wash at the sink.

I had so many tasks to complete the consultant and Hayley were pushing for discharge. I had to catheterize a patient Amber in the side room, I had to set up a drip for Thomas, and complete the discharge plan for Claude. My patient Mick was waiting for discharge as the doctors assessed that he was safe for discharge. As I completed the tasks Mick would constantly press the buzzer, "Excuse me squire, can I have a cup of tea? Can I move to a quieter bay?" he asked at times I felt like a hotel attendant, not a nurse. I managed to get through the difficult shift with the help of Sister Jackie and Jane, the hard-working healthcare assistant.

Nearing the end of the shift I heard two loud screams at the nurse's station. It was Hayley, Gill had thrown two jugs of water over her from the housekeeper's trolley. Hayley looked mortified as her donuts were now soaked. I started to laugh with Jackie and Jane. It was the perfect end to a whirlwind shift.

That evening it felt great to ride back home on my break, it was a beautiful windy summer's evening. It was the first time I had rode my bike in over five years. Then disaster when a lorry driver angrily beeped his horn, causing me to crash my bike into a bush and I flew into the hedge. I was so thankful when a young couple helped carry me out, even with the pandemic restrictions I was thankful that people were there to help.

I walked home with my flat tire, covered in bruises, I was tired and exhausted, and ready to jump into my bed and escape. As I reached my home I looked on in shock, as my Father sat at the table crying whilst looking through a photo album. My mother appeared shaking.

"What's wrong?" I asked.

"It's your uncle William, he has passed away, he died from a heart attack. William's daughter dropped this photo album off, he was planning to travel to us on Christmas day."

I sat down on the couch and began to cry.

Chapter 11: Look to the future

As I arrived at the nurse manager's office the next day, I was now excited to work on the medical ward after spending a limited time in the community. I arrived at the medical assessment ward at 7:30 am and could feel how stressed the staff were as we all sat in our masks and visas, stressed about the news reports and the news that two nurses had already called in sick. In the shift, I worked alongside sister Jackie, a fifty-year-old nurse, with over thirty years of experience on the ward. I also worked with Donald, a forty-year-old nurse from Italy who would often compliment the beautiful nurses he worked with. Then there was Alberton, one of the laziest nurses I had ever worked with. Alberton would constantly ask other nurses to complete her medication rounds and dressings, so she could enjoy time in the smoking shelter with her boyfriend.

I then met the patients I was looking after in A bay. The first patient was Albert, an eighty-year-old man admitted with confusion following his carers, found him flooding his kitchen after leaving the washing machine overnight. The second patient was George, a sixty-four-year-old ex-footballer admitted with following an infection in his leg and worsening arthritis. The third patient was Anthony who was admitted following a routine GP appointment, in which his blood pressure and blood sugar proved to be erratic and he complained about fainting episodes at home.

The final patient I was to look after was Simon, an eighty-six-year-old admitted following a worsening of his dementia condition in the care home, and the staff had stated that they struggled to cope with the change in behavior.

In the shift, I was working alongside Elizabeth, an experienced healthcare assistant, who retired after being a midwife for over fifty years. I also worked alongside a third-year student nurse called Lucy, who was hard working and motivated.

As I completed the medication round, I observed how hard-working and conscientious was being able to remember the uses and side effects of all medications. Lucy was able to encourage Simon who was reluctant to take his medication, to take them, and encouraged him to partake in his wash and dressing activity, as he actively refused to wash for three days. I then observed as Lucy and Elizabeth prepared the washing materials for each patient and provided kindness and compassion to each patient they cared for. It was so tough for Lucy and other students working as student nurses during the pandemic. Lucy worked each shift without getting paid and sacrificed her life with her children by working four twelve-hour shifts a week.

I then completed my ward round with the consultant doctor Tanzier. I had worked with doctor Tanzier on other wards as a nurse, he was renowned for her temper tantrums and angry outbursts, shouting at staff and throwing folders on the floor. Suddenly I found Doctor Tanzier shouting random instructions to me, complete bloods for Albert, encourage physio support for George, complete a blood and urine test for Anthony, and get the mental health assessment to assess Simon's current condition.
"How are you doctor Tanzier?" I asked.
"If you must know I am very unhappy Chris, for thirty years I worked in this hospital, and I have just heard that they might be closing this ward and relocating us, they are hoping to turn the hospital into a cancer-free hospital which can undertake elective surgery." he sighed.

I was in shock that so many wards were being closed due to the panic. I could see the fear and upset in the Nurse's face as they attempted to comprehend the upsetting news. As I returned to the ward, I observed that Lucy had already completed the morning observations and had now started to fill out the care plans. I then heard a loud scream in the side room. A woman walked out of the side room in anger, "Excuse me this man is in my mother's room and he is rushing to get off of her bed." I walked into the side room and observed Jean who was recovering from complications in her hip surgery. Albert was sitting on her bed, with his legs crossed reading a magazine.

"Excuse me sir do you not realize that there is a pandemic going on, get him off my bed nurse or I will scream!" she warned.

"Albert, can I talk to you in private please?"

"Ok," he smiled.

I walked alongside Albert and he was very unsteady on his Zimmer frame.

"Well, Albert you certainly are active for a Monday morning!"

"Monday? it's not Monday," he groaned.

"It is," I smiled.

I watched as Albert's face filled red with anger and rage as he threw his frame into the wall and grabbed onto my shoulders.

"You bastard! Who do you think you are lying to me? It is Sunday today. Why am I here?" he raged.

I watched as Albert became unsteady and his legs started to buckle. I shouted for help and observed Elizabeth and Lucy rushing to the scene. Lucy grabbed a pillow to protect Albert from his head and hit the floor, whilst Elizabeth wrapped her arms at a distance to protect his upper body.

We were able to successfully lower Albert to the ground, we then slowly hoisted him into his rise and recliner chair. I placed an alarm mat underneath Albert, which would alert the staff if ever he stood up to help protect him. I advised Elizabeth to stay in the bay at all times to observe Albert, as his behavior was starting to get more erratic. An hour later I received the urine and blood results and after the doctor assessed him it was confirmed that Albert had a urinary tract infection. I had looked after so many patients who developed a UTI infection, and their behavior would often completely change. Many patients would appear confused, aggressive, and many family members reported a complete change in their relative's personality.

I observed George screaming out in pain, and the tissue viability nurse assessed that he required a new dressing for his right leg. The doctor had also requested an appointment at the outpatient clinic to complete a biopsy, as he was concerned with the ongoing pain he was having in his leg. I completed the dressing and observed how upset George was, "do you know I was a professional footballer since the age of sixteen, and I have been so physically active my entire life. Not being able to move, having to use a walking stick to go everywhere, has left me completely depressed. I can't go on anymore," he cried.

"George it is a very hard time for you, it is difficult for all of us during the pandemic, but the doctor is looking to complete more investigations to examine the lump on your leg. If you need anything or anyone to speak to you, I am here for you George." I smiled.

"Thank you, Chris, it is nice to be spoken to as a human being, you show an interest in people and I admire that, you certainly are in the right job," he smiled.

I wanted to believe I was in the right job, but for so many years I was struggling with my ambition to perform in the theatre, and with my love of working in the ward as a nurse. Receiving positive feedback from George made my role as a nurse worth life, it gave me a purpose.

I then sat next to Anthony; Anthony explained that his fainting episodes started after he left his job as a headteacher. Anthony experienced stress when his school received a low grade from Ofsted and a requiring improvement grade. At the age of forty, Anthony took on the role of headteacher as an exciting challenge. However, Anthony explained that he started school when there were many pre-existing problems already in school. There was a strong culture of bullying in the school, the previous headteacher had sacked teachers he believed undermined him, and staff reported that he sacked teachers for simply disliking them.

Anthony expressed that he found the pressure so hard and he struggled to sleep, he kept on getting severe headaches, culminating in him collapsing in the staffroom. It was so difficult to see how much the stress had affected Anthony.

Anthony expressed that he found it difficult in lockdown, as his wife had left him following his unemployment.

Simon who was living with dementia was sleeping for the entire morning, he had been up all night, spending three hours standing by the entrance door attempting to break out. Simon believed that he was being held captive and would consistently hot out at staff throughout the entire shift.

I noticed during the shift in the medical ward how people were now becoming more receptive in following the covid guidelines. The visitors of the patients on the ward appeared to accept that visiting was restricted, and only granted for patients who were at the palliative stage of their illness.

I was so happy to finally go on my break; I had my usual lunch meal crackers and cheese with a refreshing irn bru drink. I observed Lucy laying across the sofa, she had red marks on her face from wearing the mask all day, she looked visibly exhausted.

"Are you ok Lucy? you have helped me so much this morning, but you seem stressed," I questioned.

"I'm just finding it hard keeping up with the demands and assessments for my course whilst working these long shifts. At the weekends my ex-partner looks after my children and I work one day a week at Mark's and Spencer's. I'm struggling to get by. I can't sleep!" She replied.

"You will get there Lucy, the third year is the most challenging year in your training, make a timetable, drink plenty, and most of all make time for yourself. You need to take a break. Would it be possible for you to take a break from your part-time job until your placement finishes?"

"I can't as a single parent I need to pay the bills and with no bursary, I have no choice," Lucy warned. I felt upset for Lucy and the other students I supported who found they had no choice but to work alongside their current student nurse duties, whilst not receiving any financial incentives for working on the frontline in the pandemic.

After our break, we returned to the ward to hear the emergency buzzer which Elizabeth had pressed. George was unresponsive in his bed and Elizabeth had already begun CPR, Lucy grabbed the crash trolley and I rushed towards George and felt the surge of adrenaline running through me. Staff from other departments charged onto the ward to help. The lead resuscitation nurse stood over me shouting instructions, as I completed the compressions.

"Go deeper, go slower, now use the mask," he shouted.

I could feel my heart tremble and my face was red with fear. During each cardiac arrest, I almost felt like a robot, focusing on everything we were taught in our training. All the staff would try thirty compressions each before inserting the face mask. I watched as the staff tirelessly completed the compressions. George passed away at 4 pm that afternoon. I went into the staffroom and broke down in tears, I wanted so much to help George, I had witnessed how much pain he was in following the infection in his leg.

Moments later as if a bolt of lightning had hit Simon as he jumped out of his bed, quickly wrapping up his belongings into his satchel and proceeded to walk with his frame along the corridor.
"Where are you going, Simon?" I asked.
"I need to get to work, I start at 9 am I work as a mechanic. I was actually meant to start five minutes ago."
I alerted the nurse in A bay Sandra to keep an eye on Simon, it was important to allow him to walk freely on the ward. To stop a person living with dementia on the ward from completing a task can increase agitation. I observed the ward clerk offering to make Simon a cup of tea, and he appeared compliant as he sat down, and Mary asked him questions about his time of being a soldier.

I then went back to my bay and completed the observations on my patients Albert and Anthony, Albert was much more settled after the ward doctor had adjusted the medication he was taking.

I then went over to Anthony and discovered that he was dressed in his home clothes and had his bag packed.

"Anthony where are you going? Are you going out for a walk?" I asked.

"Look Chris I'm really thankful for your help but I can't wait anymore, I just want to go home. I don't care what the results are of my scan, I just want to be by myself," he warned.

I could not make Anthony stay as he had the capacity to make his own decisions.

As Anthony left, Simon suddenly burst into a fit of rage. Simon grabbed all the folders by the nurse station and threw them into the air causing hundreds of pieces of paper to fly into the air. Simon then grabbed a wet floor sign and expressed that we all need to take cover. Simon was having a vivid hallucination, and it is always so important not to disregard a person's hallucination, it is important to listen attentively. Simon believed we were under attack by the opposing army.

"Simon, we need to go into the room down the corridor, we will be safe in that room," I smiled.

Simon walked nervously with his frame, as we reached his bedside he jumped onto his bed. I observed the fear and terror in his face, "It's so scary the soldiers were chasing towards me General Martin was leading the battle."

"It is all over now, I am here with you," I smiled, pulling Martin's blanket over him.

At the end of the shift senior consultant, Dr Bennet handed out ice creams to all the team for our hard work throughout the shift. Dr Bennet stood at the entrance of the ward door delivering his speech.

"I have worked in this hospital for over forty years, in various wards and the past couple of months have been the most challenging time of my career. I want to thank you all for your bravery, your hard work and commitment to your role during this hard time. You must all remember to look after your own health and take plenty of breaks. Thank you again for your help as I start my new role tomorrow.

I was exhausted that night as I walked home. I wondered how long I would need to work in the UK before returning to New York in my role as a doctor. I missed performing to crowds, and I missed being able to pursue my leisure pursuits.

Chapter 12:The calm before the storm.

Following on from the chaotic shift I enjoyed working at the eye clinic and being given an opportunity to work night shifts in order to break the monotony of day shifts. The lockdown rules had finally eased, and we were now able to visit shops, go to restaurants but wear masks inside, and go out for unlimited exercise. Now I had to adjust to a new way of life following signs on the floor in shops in order to maintain social distance, queuing up outside to grab a coffee, and talking to my neighbors on my doorstep.

I was able to gain a block booking shift at the eye clinic due to a staff member who had to take emergency leave. The eye clinic was usually a thriving busy environment, with over fifty patients waiting in the waiting area since lockdown the department was forced to close.

I was placed in a single room, with an eye test board for me to complete visual field tests, eye drops, and folders of the patients due in.

I was working in the department with Masapora, a very overpowering and interfering nurse who I worked alongside as a student nurse. Masapora stormed into the room, she slammed the door causing the floor to shudder.

"Good morning Chris, how are you, are you sure you will be ok to work on your own today?"

"Yes Masapora, I have been a nurse for a few years now."

"Well, if you need any help please contact me. I will come into check on you." she smiled. As a student Masapora was a very overpowering mentor, often checking my observations several times, constantly asking questions, and always referred to me as a student. I was working alongside Jennifer, the healthcare assistant, who would provide several cups of tea and biscuits to me throughout the day.

My first patient was John, an eighty-nine-year-old man dressed in a pea-green suit. John looked so happy to see me explaining it had been three months since he had seen anyone. "I have really struggled during the lockdown, just before March my Wife Alsa was admitted to a care home, now the only contact we have is through a glass screen. We have been married for sixty years and now I feel she's slipping away from me," John cried, in desperation, feeling guilty for his tears.

" You have to stay strong, this will not last forever!" I promised. It was clear to see how loneliness was a common theme in elderly people during the lockdown, and it was so difficult to see how radically people's lives had changed. As I turned off the lights for the visual field test, I noticed that John was making up the letters, he was concerned that his eyesight had radically deteriorated.

The next patient was Jethrey, my old friend from school, who was now a successful accountant and owned his own business. "My goodness Chris it's been so long since I've seen you, I never had the chance to tell you, but I'm so sorry for the loss of your brother."

"Well it's been eight years, but it never gets easier, I have missed him so much during the lockdown. I completed Jethreys visual field test and noticed that his eyesight remained unchanged, Jethrey had been diagnosed with type 2 diabetes. Jethrey showed me the picture of his wife and children and his beautiful mansion in the countryside. Looking at Jethrey's photo made me feel I had so much more to achieve in life.

The next patient was Lucile, a ninety-two-year-old lady with early-stage dementia, who had struggled to administer her eye drops, and required patient education.

"Mrs. Lucile Good morning how are you today?"

"Let's not talk, let's just get this over with. I hate putting in my eye drops!" she screamed. Lucile sat angrily in the swivel chair and spun around angrily.

"Well Lucile, first of all, can you show me how you put in your eye drops?" I watched as Lucile tilted her head back and proceeded to put the eye drops over her forehead and cheeks with her eyes tightly closed.

"Lucile you have to open your eyes to put your eye drops. Can we try it very slowly, I asked. I made sure Lucile was comfortable in the chair and she managed to open her eyes wide. I administered the eye drops, and all of a sudden Lucile let out a terrifying scream.

"Jesus Mary and Joseph and all the saints above in heaven, I'm blind!" she screamed. I jumped back in shock. Suddenly Masapora stormed in, "What is going on? It sounds like a cat is being thrown into the lake?" she strained. Masapora always had a way with words. After ten minutes we managed to help Lucile remain calm in the chair, and referred her to the doctor, to look at getting the carers to train to administer the eye drops.

The final patient was Jackie, a seventy-five-year-old lady requiring a visual field test. Jackie was very emotional in the confrontation explaining that she lives in a remote countryside, I can't see my family members, I can't use face apps or technology, so I really struggle!" she exclaimed. After the visual field test, Jackie carried on talking about her life in the cottage and how her Labrador Rory was her savior, her only contact. I enjoyed working at the eye clinic, unlike the ward and community environment I was able to offer one to one support to people, including emotional support.

Jenny made me several cups of tea in the shift, during each consultation I observed Masapora peeking through the door, making me feel like an eternal student. At the end of the shift Masapora walked in smiling falsely, "Well done Chris, you really did today, maybe you could come back in a few years when you gain more confidence.

After the shift, I climbed into my polo car and as I reversed back, I hit into a BMW car, the car belonged to Masapora, I collapsed into a heap in my car.

The following day I prepared for my night shift, I rarely completed night shifts even as a student. I found it difficult staying alert and would feel physically sick the following day, collapsing into a deep state of exhaustion. For my nightshift, I had prepared my crackers and cheese, my iPod filled with chill-out songs, and my toothbrush and toothpaste. I always found that brushing my teeth on my break helped me feel more awake!

I became disheartened during the day before my night shift, it was positive to observe overall cases decline, but there were still so many areas of society affected by the pandemic. Family members campaigned to the government to visit their relatives with no response, the needs of people with dementia were not addressed, and so many children were left devastated following the news that they were not being permitted to sit their exams.

In many ways, I was lucky that I had a job, a place to stay and a supportive family unit. I was more concerned for the future, I wanted financial security, my own home, and to see the world.

That evening, at 7 pm I arrived at the Alpen cardiac ward. I was working alongside Amalda, an agency nurse who would often take extended smoking breaks and would send up her camp bed and oversleep on her breaks! I was also working with Leanne, a nurse from the Philippines with over twenty years of experience. Leanne would strive to help all the nurses in the ward complete tasks and took on extra work to help others. Many of the nurses I worked within the Philippines went through a rigorous training programme which involved one to one training. I also worked with Norma, a sixty-year-old nurse who had worked on the ward for over forty years.

In the night shift, I was looking after patients between two bays which I found very difficult, especially when patients required one to one care amongst short staff levels. In the first bay, I was looking after Mary who was admitted with an exacerbation in her asthma and was also living with dementia. Mary was very physically and verbally aggressive and did not want to sleep. Next to Mary was Lucy, a fifty-year-old headteacher awaiting valve repair surgery and was struggling to rest due to the high levels of noise. Opposite Luce was Elma, a one-hundred-year-old lady and former matron of Aspen ward, Elma was in the palliative stage of her cancer condition and was supported by her devoted son Mark.

I was also supporting the two patients in A bay, Benny, a sixty-five-year-old man, admitted with sepsis. Barry was a previous army medic and enjoyed supporting all the patients on the ward. Next to Barry was Richard a seventy-two-year-old man who presented with a UTI and required one to one supervision.

I set up my folders and bed plans in the female bay, and observed the nurses rushing around the ward.

Mary began to shout at me, "Who are you and why are you wearing a mask?"

"I'm a nurse, I'm here to look after you, I'm wearing a mask to help prevent germs from spreading!" I answered

"I don't want to go to bed, I want to go home!" Mary shouted, Suddenly Mary let out a roaring scream and the nurses explained that Mary shouted frequently during the day, but due to her dementia she really struggled.

"Please can I go to a side room, I really need to sleep, I had my operation tomorrow," Lucy explained.

"There are two people in the side rooms already when they are free, I will notify you," I explained, I observed the anguish on Lucy's face.

I then walked towards Elma's bed space and along with the healthcare assistants Leanne and Norma, we helped to reposition her in the bed. Mark explained that Elma had worked on the Aspen ward from the age of eighteen and trained over one hundred nurses, she worked as a midwife, and later trained to be a CPR expert practitioner, conducting groundbreaking research.

I then walked into the male bay to check on Barry and Richard. Barry had recovered after contracting the life-threatening sepsis condition. Barry would complete his own care plans, make his own hospital bed, and tidy up his own bed space. Barry explained that he was a dedicated medic in the army for twenty years and was specialized in completing wound care. After he left the army, he became a medical researcher.

I then observed Richard sitting in his chair angrily with his pants over his trousers holding a stick in his hand.

"Get away from me, I don't want you to go near me!" he shouted. Richard believed he was in prison, and his UTI infection had worsened his mental state. As an experienced nurse, I witnessed that the ward environment including lights, noise, and furniture arrangement all affected patients. Irene looked physically exhausted.

"This is my fifth night shift in a row, two staff members are in isolation, and I have been asked to cover. I am constantly drinking coffee, I have to isolate myself from my husband, it is so stressful," she explained. I made sure Irene took plenty of breaks throughout the shift to prevent burn out. I observed that nurses were being stretched to their limits.

For the remainder of the shift I felt fully supported by my colleagues, and all my patients were all medically stable. Mary became more and more agitated, so Lucy decided to sit outside the bay listening to her meditation app.

At 5pm, I could hear Irene shouting for help. Suddenly we all rushed in, Richard managed to lock himself in the bathroom. At first, he began to smash items in the bathroom with his walking stick. He then ran the bath causing a flood to occur in the bay. We called the security team, and when they opened the door the water nearly drowned us, as we observed Richard in the bathtub in his clothes. We arranged for a mental health nurse to sit with him and for further assessment the next day with the crisis team. It was a very stressful night shift, but the support from the staff helped me to get through.

The following day, whilst my parents went for a walk in the countryside, Harry helped me to set up decorations for a small celebration for my parent's fortieth wedding anniversary. I baked a cake, and Harry helped to decorate the table with a part that's confetti, whilst I placed finger food on the table. It was wonderful to be able to spend time together. Before they arrived, my Sister Louise knocked on the door, holding a neatly wrapped present.

"Before you ask, I've had a negative test and I just need to get away from my friend for a while," she warned. I watched as Louise draped herself on the sofa, "by the way please don't tell Mum and Dad what happened," she warned. When my parents returned, they were delighted and perplexed at Louise's secret return. Louise was mysterious like my brother Michael; they were both impulsive, there was so much Louise kept hidden. That afternoon we danced, sang, and enjoyed looking through past photo albums. It would be the final time we would spend all together in our childhood home.

The following few weeks were difficult, my parents had finally sold their house, and Harry had to be isolated at home due to a child testing positive for the virus. I finally had to say goodbye to my childhood home. I spent hours packing up Michael's belongings including his clothes, books, textbooks and written letters. I then discovered an extensive journal he had written during his time as a doctor. I found it so difficult. Every part of our childhood home reminded me of Michael. On the tree outside we carved our names on the floorboard, on the pavement in the garden, we imprinted our hands on our 10th birthday. We shared so many memories in the house. We had parties with our friends whilst our parents went on holiday. I comforted Michael during his cancer battle in our room each night. At nighttime, we would sit by our window ledge talking about our hopes and future dreams, whilst studying for our dreams.

On my final afternoon, I was very tearful as I sat in the garden with my Mum. "I know the past few months have been very difficult for you, I know you miss your acting roles."
"I miss it, but I know that the pandemic is temporary, and the situation has affected us all. I'm sure going to miss this house, but it's time for us all to move on and look to the future. For the first time in my life, I have no plan

and that is how I will leave in 2020, but now I realize that my friends and family are the most important aspect of my life.

On my final day in the house, I prepared a time capsule with Harry to bury our memories of 2020, and our hopes for the future. In Harry's box, he placed his drawings of the rainbows and 'save NHS' posters he created. In my box, I wrote a letter explaining my life with my brother in my house, my hopes for the future as a nurse, and an account of the battle I faced during 2020. As we stood outside the house that afternoon ready to go to our temporary apartment, I cried, and finally said goodbye to my past. With no plan for the future, we drove off in my Father's car, and I knew for the first time I was finally moving on.

Chapter 13: Reflection for the future.

2020 has been one of the most challenging years we have all faced, it has been so difficult having to isolate from family, friends and give up our hobbies and interests. In the hospital, as nurses, we faced challenges and stretched more than we could imagine. We have had to work twelve-hour shifts, wearing masks under short staffing levels, heightened pressure, and escalated fear of patients and staff alike.

We have looked after patients with coronavirus and observed the devastating effects of the virus on the most vulnerable in society.

Throughout the pandemic, I have cried at the end of a shift, collapsed into a chair, exhausted from the long shift.

It has been so difficult returning home and having to isolate and maintain social distance from my own family members. There have been numerous times I wished I could return to New York, and hideout in my apartment and escape the realities of the real world.

However, despite the many negative consequences of the pandemic. I have also witnessed the kindness of humans and support for the NHS. I marveled at the clapping every Thursday, and the appreciation for the

NHS. I have observed people giving to charities and food banks, and I have watched my colleagues work together, to provide patient-centered care and continue to fight our battle.

Chapter 14: A letter from my brother.

Dear Chris, I want to thank you for all your support over the past couple of years with my cancer battle. You have really helped to keep me positive during the darkest of my days. Although we know I am close to losing this battle, I want to tell you my hopes for you in the future and I have left a few surprises for you. Hidden in the house are money and gifts I have left to help you all in the future.

I want you to stay strong in the future and lead the life you dream of. For so long now you have focused on your studies and career but have not focused on making friends or having fun. Make sure you continue to travel, make opportunities to travel, speak to strangers, and know that wherever you are I will always be guiding you forever.

I have written a journal of my time as a doctor which I feel can help others in the future, please share it with my hospital colleagues and Mum and Dad, it explains so much about my life that I've kept hidden.

I want to thank you for being the best brother I could ask for. You have given me a great life, and please don't forget the difference you have made to me and others you have cared for.

I'll always be here for you always, Michael.

Chapter 15: Top tips for a nurse post-2020

Make sure you take plenty of time to rest, make sure you get over eight hours of sleep a night. If you feel stressed or are finding it difficult to sleep, use scented candles, or listen to relax music to help you unwind each day.

After a long shift make sure you undertake thirty minutes of exercise each day, dancing, running, or participating in yoga can help you feel relaxed, rescue stress and elevate your mood.

Reach out to friends who you feel may be struggling during the pandemic, phoning a friend or getting in touch with someone you haven't spoken to in years. You could make a difference.

If you are completing essays or assessments make sure you take plenty of breaks on your day off, going for a brisk walk in between studying can help consolidate what you have learnt. When studying try to create a written timetable and stick to it.

If you are part of a union or a forum at the hospital seek support from your peers, who are struggling at this time, someone could be waiting for your advice and support.

Make sure you bring your lunch every day on shift and drink plenty of water. It is vital to eat and drink to give you energy and to help you to function fully during the shift.

Keep a diary of three positive things you have achieved each shift, it is important to remain positive and focus on good practice.

Use your time off and free days in lockdown to be creative. Drawing, painting and writing your memoir can be very therapeutic and help you to consolidate negative feelings. I have found writing my experiences down on paper as being the best therapy I could have, to overcome negative experiences.

After each shift try to keep a reflective journal it is so important to reflect on how we can improve following each shift.

Never be afraid to challenge people or other staff members in the hospital, who are not following social distancing rules, it is everyone's role to protect ourselves and others during the pandemic.

Working on the ward can be both physically and emotionally draining during these difficult times. If you feel you're too depressed to work, ask for a time out, and take your annual leave when you can.

Always be kind and patient to student nurses they are training during one of the most challenging times and will need time to learn, adjust, and comprehend the demands of nursing. If you are a mentor, hold weekly meetings with your student nurse, to reflect on their progress and to have a chance to talk about what they have found difficult. Encourage students to attend student forums, and gain support from their university peers.

Support elderly people in the community by helping those who are immobile by offering help with shopping, you could make a big impact to a person's life.

It is important during these challenging times to keep a record of your finances and spending. Keeping a weekly and monthly budget can help you, avoid unnecessary spending if possible.

So many people have lost their jobs during the pandemic and offer your support to friends requiring support in looking for a job. Reading over an application form, notifying a friend of job openings, and holding a mock interview could really make a difference to a friend who is struggling.

Remember there's always hope for a better day and what we are all going through now is only temporary.

If you have recently moved to a new area and are struggling to connect with others try to join a local online community, online quizzes and groups can be a great way to connect with others.

To try to boost your own morale it may help you to avoid the number of news articles or reports you read. If you feel affected by the pandemic news articles, try to limit yourself to only accessing essential news articles or briefings.

Look after your hands moisturize them and bathe your hands in hot soapy water at home to try and heal your hands if you have to frequently wash them due to your role.

Try to understand that the staff members you are working with maybe going through personal struggles at home, if you know your colleagues are struggling to offer a friendly ear. If you feel your colleagues need space, give them space.

We must stick together and remember why we became nurses, keeping our core values of kindness, compassion and care at the heart of everything we do.

I want to thank the staff at the University Hospital Birmingham Trust and Yorkshire hospital trusts for all your support.

I want to thank all my family for their continued support.

Thank you to the fantastic cover designer of my book Scott Gaunt, your covers help bring my books to life!

If you enjoy my book, please leave a review. For future updates or to get in contact please follow me on instagram @buttinchris or on twitter @christo25288316

The end.

www.ingramcontent.com/pod-product-compliance
Lightning Source LLC
Chambersburg PA
CBHW070643220526
45466CB00001B/275